BEHIND BULLETPROOF GLASS

MY STORY ABOUT PRENATAL TESTING AND ABORTION IN THE UNITED STATES

LINDA RÖNN

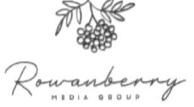

Rowanberry
MEDIA GROUP

TO MY DAUGHTER

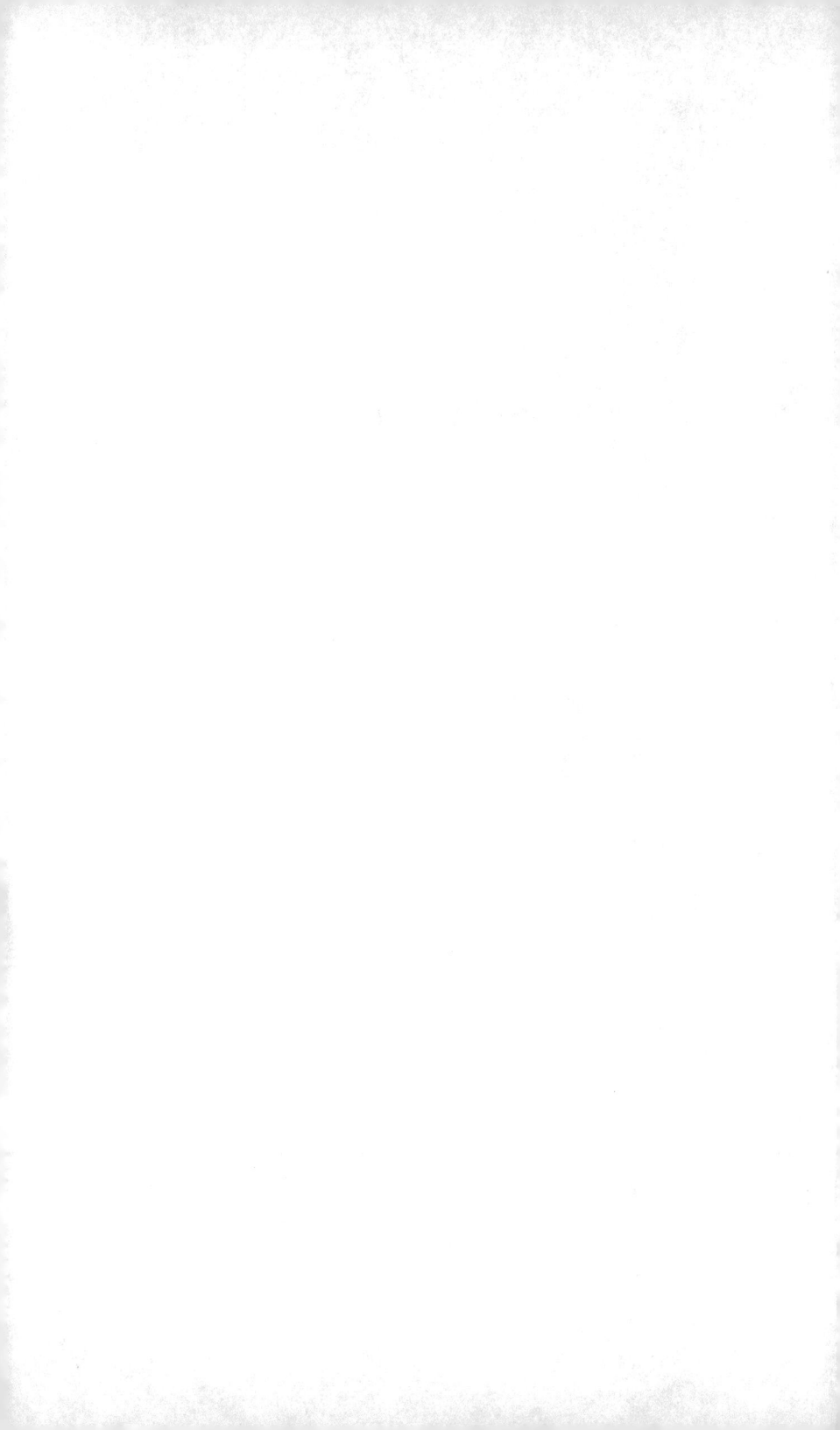

The angel, in the book of life
Wrote down my baby's birth
And whispered as she closed the book
"Too beautiful for earth."

— UNKNOWN

PROLOGUE

I woke up with a knot in my stomach. The dreaded day had finally arrived. Our appointment at Planned Parenthood was scheduled for after lunch. Despite my desire to get it over with, I didn't want to go. I clutched my phone and searched for information on abortion procedures, recovery, and potential risks. Google was a blessing and a curse.

Juni was already at preschool, and we dropped off our Brittany, Leia, at the doggie daycare on our way to the abortion clinic. A security guard was standing in front of the building, and he pointed us to a hidden parking lot in the back. There were no protesters outside, but the security guard's presence didn't put me at ease. Why was he standing there?

The security guard nodded at us as we walked around the building to the entrance. I wore my most comfortable clothes—yoga pants, a stretchy tank top, and a sweatshirt. We went inside, and the brutality of American reality struck me when I saw the receptionist sitting shielded behind bulletproof glass. She checked my driver's license before she pushed a button to let us into the waiting room, hidden behind a locked door. I walked up to the next window, where another receptionist was also sitting behind bulletproof glass. I spoke with her through a handset, which reminded me of prison visits I had seen in movies. The security measures were overwhelming. I paid the 300-dollar copay—my health insurance covered the rest—and signed a few documents before they asked us to sit down and wait.

The waiting room was spacious; the blinds were closed tight, blocking the view in and out. A few other patients were already sitting in the room. No one made eye contact with us. Magazines lay scattered on the tables, and the movie *The Holiday*, starring Cameron Diaz and Kate Winslet, was playing on a TV screen. Posters asking for donations covered the walls. They reminded us that Planned Parenthood wouldn't receive any tax funds if President Donald Trump and the Republicans got their way.

How did I end up here?

I was excited when I found out I was pregnant with our second child—I looked forward to a happy ending and a bigger family. But that didn't happen. Life took a turn I never could have expected.

The prenatal testing results revealed the fetus had a chromosomal abnormality. The number of abortions performed because of medical reasons is small, considering the wide range of reasons people choose the procedure. These women want children but choose to have an abortion with the best interest of the fetus and the family in mind. I was one of those women.

I loved the life that was growing inside my body. I loved it so much that I had an abortion. Maybe I couldn't give it life, but I could give it peace. I could let its heart stop beating while it was safe inside me. That other people should have anything to do with our decision was unimaginable, but that was the cruel reality.

One in four pregnancies in Sweden end in abortion, and one in four women in the United States will have an abortion before turning forty-five. Despite this, we rarely hear women's voices on the matter. Society stigmatizes the decision, and it's considered taboo for women to talk about their experiences. And yet, American news channels discuss abortion rights almost daily.

A multitude of factors affect how you experience your abortion—where in the world you live, your culture, class, religious beliefs, personal circumstances, life experience, and the opinions of the people around you. But they all have one thing in common. If you choose to have an abortion, you're forced to justify or explain your decision in a way that few other situations demand. The stigmatization against abortion is deeply ingrained in society, which results in shame that prevents us from speaking of it. This silence reinforces the stigmatization.

It's imperative for us to break this vicious circle of stigma, shame, and silence, and to do so, we must talk about abortions. Our stories must be told, and they must be heard.

So, here's my story.

My journey didn't begin in a sterile and hidden waiting room. As for many others, it all started much earlier.

1

A SECOND CHILD

I was eighteen years old when I first came to the United States. A few months earlier, I had graduated from high school. I was unsure of my future, so when a friend told me she planned to work as an au pair in the United States, I jumped at the opportunity to join her. The gap year would give me time to decide what to do next. It wasn't until I received the letter about my assigned family living in Maryland that I learned it was a state in America.

I spent a year on the East Coast, in a suburb outside Washington, DC, before I returned to my parents in southern Sweden for a visit. After the holidays, I packed my bags again and headed north to study at Uppsala University. A semester later, I couldn't resist the pull toward the West, so I returned to the United States to attend a university in San Diego. After graduating with a bachelor of arts degree in international security & conflict resolution and an MBA in marketing a few years later, I stayed.

My husband, John, grew up in Washington, DC, just a few minutes' drive from the family I lived with as an au pair. He joined the Navy after college and served as an officer for a few years. His final assignment was in San Diego, and he also stayed in the city.

We met in 2007 at RT's Longboard Grill in Pacific Beach. Our dog Leia joined the family in 2008; in 2011, we got married overlooking the Pacific Ocean. Our daughter Juni was born a few years later. We were lucky to have a healthy daughter and loved her more than anything.

We lived less than a mile from the beach, and I understood why San Diego is called America's Finest City. We loved the mild climate and the many opportunities for outdoor activities. I missed things about Sweden, particularly when I thought about the differences in government and politics. I believe all children should get free school lunches, that everyone should have healthcare coverage, and that laws should limit access to guns. Many Americans disagreed with me, which became evident in conversations with coworkers and acquaintances. But politics aside, I enjoyed our life here.

We had just welcomed the new year in 2017 when I noticed my period was a few days late. John and I waited anxiously for the pregnancy test to reveal the result. We felt a mix of emotions when we saw it was positive. We were excited, as we had talked about having a second child, but also a little nervous. Juni, our daughter, was two and a half years old, and the age difference between siblings felt right.

John had recently lost his full-time job as a project manager for an industrial software company because the company had decided to close its San Diego office. They offered him a remote, part-time position for a few months, and he accepted it since we knew it could take a while to find a new job, but our future financial situation was uncertain. And, while our house was perfect for our current family, it would be tight with a new addition.

The pregnancy motivated John to search for a new job, and

we started planning renovations for our house to fit our growing family better. We were confident that all the pieces would fall into place. We shared the joyous news with our close friends and family, and my parents planned to visit us after the baby's arrival. I downloaded a pregnancy tracking app on my phone and started the countdown to the due date. We looked forward to fall when the baby would arrive.

The pregnancy was challenging—like my first. The relentless nausea, sometimes to the point of vomiting, was crippling. I knew from experience that eating crackers and drinking ginger ale wouldn't help me. The medication my doctor had recommended for the nausea didn't work, and the pregnancy was wearing me down. I was exhausted and downhearted, but I didn't think anything would go wrong. I didn't enjoy being pregnant, but the pregnancy wouldn't last forever.

I couldn't understand how some women loved being pregnant and even missed it afterward. I experienced my first pregnancy as an uncomfortable but necessary journey until Juni was born. Breastfeeding was painful and anxiety-provoking, so I only breastfed her for a few months. Many critics think breastfeeding should last longer, but it didn't harm her. People have opinions about everything regarding pregnancy, breastfeeding, and child-rearing.

I went back to work full time as a data analyst for a medical group when Juni was six months old, since parental leave in the United States leaves much to be desired. I was fortunate to work for a company that permitted me to take much time off from work. John's parental leave only lasted two weeks, which was too short. But we were grateful that we found a childcare center and preschool that we all loved. The waiting list spoke volumes, and we were fortunate to secure a spot.

I decided not to breastfeed our second child to avoid the anxiety it gave me last time. John could shoulder more responsibilities at home so I could get the rest I needed. I also had the advantage of working from home, so I didn't have to pretend to feel well around my coworkers. Our finances were tight, but we would make it work.

But things took a turn for the worse. Donald Trump was inaugurated as President of the United States in January 2017, the same month we found out I was pregnant. And everything went downhill from there.

Back in Sweden, the year started with bad news. My mom found out that she had some cell changes, and she had to go through countless tests until her doctor scheduled surgery to remove one of her kidneys. I desperately wanted to see her but hesitated to take the long trip because of my constant nausea. I scheduled an appointment at the Swedish Consulate to renew my passport in case the situation worsened. My mom's condition made it highly doubtful that my parents could visit after the baby's arrival. It became a matter of survival instead.

Around the same time, some of my close friends were also dealing with health issues. I usually turn off the volume on my phone at night to avoid being woken up by notifications. One Sunday morning, I woke up to see several text messages from Henrik, one of my best friends. He had messaged me at one in the morning to tell me he had driven himself to the emergency room, where he had put me as his emergency contact on the intake form. A few hours later, he had sent additional messages telling me they would need to remove a gallstone.

My guilty conscience was killing me when I woke up that morning. I wish I had been able to be there for Henrik. The next afternoon, John and Eddie, my best friend Sara's husband, went to the hospital to bring Henrik some things from his house. By then, Henrik had already had a procedure done. He was supposed to be discharged and come back a few weeks later for a more extensive surgery to remove the gallbladder. But the excruciating pain returned, so on Tuesday, they performed the surgery. That Wednesday, we waited nervously to hear from him. We had heard there had been complications, and that they were keeping him sedated. What had happened? I thought it was a standard procedure. We spent Thursday waiting for updates. I received the long-awaited message during a work meeting: *I'm okay now*. He was awake. To our relief, he was discharged a few days later and could go home.

My other close friend, Jenny, became pregnant around the same time I did. Even though doctors recommend waiting to share the news with friends and family until week 12—when the risk for miscarriage decreases dramatically—we had told each other before that. We joked we should send John and her husband Matt to get vasectomies together since both of us felt that we would be done having children after this. On the day of her first doctor's appointment, I texted her to ask how it went.

It didn't cross my mind that something could be wrong.

My heart broke into a thousand pieces when she responded that the doctor hadn't been able to find a heartbeat. Blood and tears filled the following weeks. She said she was grateful she hadn't told more people about the pregnancy. My pregnancy continued as planned, but I suffered with Jenny as she grieved.

The year seemed doomed from the beginning.

2

PRENATAL TESTING

I was thirty-five years old when Juni was born, and at thirty-eight, my second pregnancy was considered a "geriatric pregnancy." We didn't hesitate to do the prenatal tests the doctor recommended, even though I thought everything would be okay. I was healthy, and I had given birth to a healthy child three years earlier. We expected the tests to confirm that the fetus was healthy, and that everything would proceed as planned.

We weren't prepared for what we would do if the tests showed the opposite.

Prenatal testing reveals chromosomal abnormalities or conditions and the fetus's sex. Some tests are screenings, like ultrasounds and Non-Invasive Prenatal Testing (NIPT), a blood test that screens for chromosomal abnormalities. Then there are diagnostic tests, such as amniocentesis, chorionic villus sampling (CVS), and, in some cases, ultrasounds. Ultrasounds are possible at any point in pregnancy, but certain tests have specific week limitations. Amniocentesis and CVS carry a slight miscarriage risk, while the other tests are safer by comparison. You don't *have* to do prenatal testing, but the options are available. The risks of chromosomal abnormalities increase with age, so doctors recommend prenatal testing if you are over thirty-five years old. Your health insurance coverage determines which tests are included.

I was younger during my first pregnancy, but I still did a nuchal translucency scan combined with a blood test, since my insurance didn't cover NIPT for members under thirty-five years old. All those tests looked good, and we learned we were expecting a daughter at the routine ultrasound in week 18.

This time, we did the NIPT since I was over thirty-five. My pregnancy was high-risk because of my age, so my health insurance covered all the necessary tests.

NIPT is a simple blood test administered after week 10 that screens for chromosomal abnormalities. Trisomy 21, also known as Down syndrome, is one of the more common variations. Still, there are many other chromosome variations. Further testing is usually unnecessary if the NIPT shows no risk of chromosome abnormalities. If the screening shows a risk, further testing is necessary to know for sure, like a CVS or amniocentesis. The NIPT results are called false positives if the additional tests conclude there are no abnormalities.

It's essential to consider a course of action if a test doesn't give you the result you had hoped for, though many don't expect any issues. Some may want to find out if there are any variations so they can prepare for the life of a child with extra needs, or they may want to have an abortion. But in the end, most people do prenatal testing expecting good news. Many say, "I don't care if it's a boy or a girl, as long as it's healthy," and want to confirm it. Some want to find out the sex, to choose a name, and maybe select the paint color for the nursery. Then, some get tested and will continue the pregnancy, no matter the result. And some people say that the result doesn't matter, that they would still proceed—yet privately plan to terminate the pregnancy.

Statistics show pregnant women are taking advantage of prenatal testing to make informed decisions. In Iceland, the impact is most evident—since prenatal testing became available, almost 100 percent of pregnant women whose fetuses are diagnosed with Down syndrome decide to have an abortion. The percentage is lower in other countries, but the trend is the same. The estimated figure in the United States is 67 percent, while in the United Kingdom, it's 90 percent. In Sweden, the number of children born with Down syndrome is decreasing—122 were born in 2016, compared to 183 in 2014. The decrease is happening even though women, on average, are older when they give birth, so the number of children with Down syndrome should increase. Increased access to prenatal testing is likely the explanation for the decrease.

The increase in prenatal testing is leading to fewer children with Down syndrome being born, which upsets some people. Some Republican politicians have even proposed an abortion ban when the sole reason for the procedure is the diagnosis of Down syndrome in the fetus. However, critics argue these bills are against the Constitution and have the intention of moving toward banning abortions altogether rather than protecting people with Down syndrome. These politicians push for restrictions without discussing increased benefits, healthcare, and other forms of support that children with Down syndrome may need.

Many organizations for parents of children with Down syndrome have avoided taking a stand regarding anti-abortion laws since opinions differ in these groups as well. Some advocate for autonomy over their pregnancies, while some are concerned about missed opportunities to become a parent. Some parents whose children didn't get the diagnosis until after birth may wonder what they would have done if they had known sooner. There are no obvious answers.

Some people criticize those who choose to have an abortion after the fetus is diagnosed with Down syndrome. They question which chromosomal abnormalities and disabilities society deems acceptable. I think each pregnant person should have the final say. No one else should be the judge. All families should be able to decide what is best for them, with or without a diagnosis. I wish the discussion would end there.

When I learned about my second pregnancy, my best friend, Sara, was already pregnant, and she was expecting a girl. Our child would be four months younger, and I already envisioned how our children would play together. Our NIPT results would reveal the sex of the fetus, and the results are usually available one to two weeks after the test. After a week, we still hadn't heard anything, but I wasn't worried, as I had a doctor's appointment scheduled less than a week later. I expected that my doctor would discuss the results then. We had shared the pregnancy news with a close circle of family members and friends. After Jenny's miscarriage, I refrained from sharing the news with others at this early stage. It bothered me when friends who knew about the pregnancy asked about the results. I felt scarred by my friend's grief and didn't want to rush any answers. We would find out soon enough.

A group of friends and I organized a baby shower for Sara and her husband, Eddie, that weekend. I struggled to hide my pregnancy from the guests. After all, I was almost at week 12 when most people shared the news. Our friend Andrew, who knew I was pregnant, approached me and asked, "How are you doing? Are you nauseous?"

Feeling nauseous, I nodded and whispered, "Please don't say anything—most people here don't know I'm pregnant." I didn't think anyone overheard our conversation or noticed I didn't sip the wine. I was busy organizing games, serving food, and watching Juni. It surprised me I was able to hide my nausea. I could have won an Oscar for my acting talent.

3

THE NIPT RESULT

The day after Sara and Eddie's baby shower, I was exhausted and decided any more social events had to wait until my nausea disappeared. I would be able to explain my avoidance soon enough.

The phone rang at 5:57 p.m. The call lasted 9 minutes and 37 seconds; it was the phone call that changed everything.

I worked for the medical group where I received my medical care, so I recognized the phone number even though it wasn't saved on my phone. It was my doctor. He barely congratulated me on the pregnancy and brushed off my complaints about my nausea. Instead, he wanted to talk about the NIPT result. It was this moment when he was supposed to say that everything looked good, that the fetus was healthy.

Dr. Robertson paused, and my heartbeat sped up. I heard him take a deep breath before he said, "I am so sorry, but the test showed that there is a risk that the fetus has a chromosomal abnormality."

I didn't understand what he meant, but the questions got stuck in my throat. He continued, "I'll send a referral to a specialist, and they should call you within the next two days."

My entire world was spinning. I could hardly hear what the doctor said about how unusual this abnormality was. I felt like I couldn't breathe. The reality of the reason for taking these tests hit me hard. We all want to hear that everything looks good. Nobody wants to hear about potential issues with the fetus. How was this possible? Sure, I was slightly old for a pregnancy, but the risks were still minimal.

I failed to ask any sensible questions. The only words I could put together into a complete sentence were: "Should we come to the appointment later this week?"

"Yes, of course you can come," he confirmed. "I'm sure you'll be searching for answers and have a lot of questions." Of course. Google has become every doctor's nightmare. Most patients look up their symptoms on the internet before they seek care.

I had walked to the upstairs bedroom to take the call since Juni was having a tea party with Leia in the living room. After hanging up, I stumbled downstairs as my tears welled up. I could barely see as I entered the kitchen and faced John.

"The doctor called. There's something wrong with the baby."

It was all I could say before I sank to the floor, sobbing.

"Wait, what do you mean?" John asked. He kneeled and wrapped his arms around me. I hyperventilated and couldn't repeat the doctor's words at first. He had said there was a risk that the fetus had a chromosomal abnormality, and it was so unusual that he had to refer us to a specialist. John vaguely remembered hearing of the diagnosis in a biology class at college. He didn't know what it meant, either.

John had picked up dinner from the Thai restaurant down the street, but the food remained untouched. Tears streamed down my face as I searched the internet for information, unsure of what to search for. I had heard of Down syndrome, but what was this other chromosomal abnormality the doctor had mentioned?

I frantically clicked through as many search results as I could find. On the Swedish National Board of Health and Welfare website, I found very little information under the heading for unusual diagnoses.

I looked over at John, who sat on the couch, scrolling his phone for answers. "Are you finding anything?" I asked. He shook his head. I didn't know if it was because he didn't find anything or because of the unreal situation. My search with English terms yielded a little more information, but not much. I read a few lines, then threw my phone to the floor in anger and frustration, tears still flowing, only to pick it back up and repeat the same procedure a few minutes later. It was impossible to understand this foreign reality life had thrust us into. Google, of course, only gave us vague answers.

"But wait a second," John exclaimed. "Is it possible there's nothing wrong with the baby? That the test result is incorrect?"

I sighed, daring to feel a flash of hope. "It could be. The doctor mentioned that as well." NIPT can't give a diagnosis—you have to take more tests to find out if the risk indication is correct. We analyzed stories of women who had initially received bad news but later discovered that their NIPT results were inaccurate through further testing. We didn't know what to think. All we knew was that the fetus had a tangible risk of a chromosomal abnormality.

We read everything we could find about chromosomal abnormalities, which are variations in the number and/or structure of the chromosomes. These variations can cause abnormalities and symptoms, like intellectual disabilities and autism. Special appearances are also common. The symptoms and severity vary, even among people with the same diagnosis. The list of possible problems was long, but the list of questions we needed answers to was even longer.

We read an article about a family in our situation who decided to terminate the pregnancy. My gut twisted when I read the comments where people accused them of murdering their child. John feared this hinted at what might await us. He speculated on what it would be like to have a family member with a chromosomal abnormality. I didn't even want to think about it. It hurt too much. I couldn't handle it.

I called Sara and told her what we had found out, and she promised not to tell anyone except Eddie. I don't even remember how we put Juni to bed that evening.

I slept restlessly, only in short increments. Each time I woke up, it only took a few seconds before I remembered that our life may have changed forever, and the tears would come flowing again.

With my mom's surgery scheduled for the following day, I knew I wouldn't be able to focus on work, so I took the day off. I spent the day on the couch sobbing and searching for more information on the internet. Before this, my knowledge of chromosomal abnormalities was minimal. I knew about Down syndrome and that it had something to do with an extra chromosome, but not much more. And it wasn't Down syndrome that our fetus possibly had; it was something I had never heard of. I read article after article, post after post. The pile of crumpled tissues grew.

We heard nothing regarding my mom's surgery, so I kept the volume on my phone on during the night so I would wake up if anyone from Sweden called or sent a message. I wouldn't make the same mistake as when Henrik was admitted to the hospital.

After another sleepless night, I sent a text message to my dad in the morning.

Have you heard anything from the hospital?

Dad called me right away. I could tell that he was upset. My mom was awake, but there had been complications during the surgery. The surgeon had cut her spleen by mistake, and her blood levels had dropped drastically, so she had needed blood transfusions.

"It's a common surgery, damn it," my dad growled. He asked how I was doing, but I couldn't tell him. I mentioned our doctor's appointment later that day and let him believe it was routine. He was going to the hospital to visit my mom later; we would talk more then. My mom called an hour later. She was exhausted, and her speech slurry, but hearing her voice was an incredible relief. I didn't tell her, either.

We sat in the doctor's waiting room at 9:40 a.m. I didn't have to leave a urine sample, which I had done on previous visits, so it was apparent that I wasn't here for a regular checkup. Dr. Robertson was late, but I knew he gave all his patients the time they needed, and I would get my time when it was my turn. He was one of the highest-rated physicians in our medical group, and I understood why. He took his time, listened, and patiently answered all questions, even in the most challenging moments.

While we waited for Dr. Robertson, the nurse called the specialty clinic I had been referred to and handed me the phone.

"Do you want to see a genetic counselor now or wait until week 16?" the woman on the other end of the line asked. Was that a serious question?

"Of course we want to see them as soon as possible," I answered. She said we could come right after the doctor's appointment.

The nurse escorted us into the exam room. I sat on the exam table, and John sat in one chair, my purse perched on the other. A knock on the door broke the silence. Dr. Robertson opened it and walked in. He ripped off the figurative Band-Aid and dove into why we were there.

"I know you are worried about the test result, but remember, it could be a false positive." His calm voice was the opposite of the wave of emotions rustling inside me.

I couldn't get any words out, so I nodded.

"Okay, let's see what we've got here." I lay down, and Dr. Robertson squirted gel across my belly. I flinched for a second; it was colder than I had expected. He moved the ultrasound wand back and forth, stopped when he found what he was looking for, and pointed to the screen.

"Look, she's waving." The sound of the heartbeat seemed to echo his words.

My stomach tightened, and the pressure on my chest seemed to push out the tears I had tried to hold back. *She.* The ultrasound didn't seem to affect John—his complete focus was on the chance it could be a false positive.

I mustered what little strength remained to have a conversation I never thought I would have. Not now, not with this pregnancy.

"I don't know how I'll feel if there's an abnormality." My voice trembled. "Abortion's not out of the question . . . I don't know. I need to find out more." The hope of a false positive was still there for me, but I needed to say it out loud. The thing I didn't want to think about, but that occupied my mind day and night.

"I understand, and please know that I support a woman's right to make decisions about her own body," Dr. Robertson reassured me. "You know, if a patient wants to have an abortion, sometimes I can do it, but I can't talk about it. If people find out about it, there's a risk people will protest outside the hospital, and the medical group wants to avoid complaints."

His statement made me question why I lived in the United States. This country isn't ideal for women facing this choice— but it was a choice I would consider. I wasn't sure if John felt the same way I did, as we hadn't properly discussed it yet. John was more conservative in college, but his time in the military during the Iraq War had changed some of his political beliefs, and he had become more liberal, even before we met.

I can't fathom being married to someone who is against abortion. When your doctor tells you he must sneak around to perform this procedure, that shows something is wrong in society—far different from Sweden's approach.

I feared they would dump us off at the specialist, so I asked: "We're going to the specialist after this. Will I only see them from now on?"

"No, I'm your doctor, and no matter what you decide, I'll be there for you. I'll continue to be your team's quarterback," he assured me—such an American expression. But I was relieved that he wouldn't disappear. I needed his calmness and wanted people around me I felt comfortable with.

"I know you're still nauseous, so I'll send a prescription to the pharmacy that may help. Also, on your way out, please book the prenatal appointments for the coming months. My calendar fills up quickly."

I appreciated his positive thinking—maybe it was a false positive, and my pregnancy would continue as planned.

We paid the parking fee and continued to the specialist's office a few minutes away by car. Other pregnant women were sitting in the waiting room, all of us there, most likely for different issues.

Typically, genetic counseling is offered when there are hereditary diseases in the family or when prenatal testing reveals that the fetus has a risk of a genetic diagnosis. Genetic counselors assess the pregnancy and family history, explain options for prenatal testing, help patients understand test results, and decide about further testing. They also provide information about the child's future care if that were to become necessary. In the United States, genetic counselors have a degree in genetics and counseling. In Sweden, they have a degree in health science (e.g., a nurse, midwife, biomedical analyst, or molecular biologist), social work, psychology, or equivalent subjects and have also passed an exam in genetic counseling.

After a while, they called our name, and we walked into the genetic counselor's office. She introduced herself as Kaori, shook our hands, and asked us to sit down. The room was hot and muggy, and I felt uncomfortable. But my nausea was the least of my problems now.

"Do you know what the test result means? Did someone inform you about the possible diagnosis?" she asked. We said that we had searched for information on the internet and talked to my doctor, but that everything was too overwhelming. We still had a lot of questions.

She explained the test result, "The probability that the NIPT result is correct is approximately 38 percent." She paused. The result wasn't definitive, but there was still a significant and concerning risk that something could be wrong. I would have liked to play the lottery with those odds.

"You can do a CVS or amniocentesis to determine if the NIPT result is correct. During the CVS, they take a sample of tissue from the placenta to test, but please keep in mind that the abnormality could exist in the placenta, not the fetus. An amniocentesis would give you a definitive answer, but that comes with a slight risk of miscarriage," Kaori continued.

"I don't want to take any chances; I need to know for sure," I said.

John squeezed my hand and said: "Yes, I agree. Let's do the amniocentesis." We wanted to find out with certainty if the risk indication from the NIPT was correct or not.

The amniocentesis procedure involves testing a sample of cells from amniotic fluid. Using a needle and ultrasound, the doctor locates a safe spot to drain fluid without harming the fetus. There's a slight risk of miscarriage, but we were willing to take that risk to get a definite answer. We would have to wait a bit longer before we could do the test because doctors typically perform amniocentesis at week 15 at the earliest.

We were disappointed to learn that the genetic counselor didn't know as much as we had hoped about the chromosomal abnormality that the fetus may have had. The variation was so rare that little research was available, even to medical professionals. It meant we faced a possible diagnosis that we, let alone doctors and scientists in the field, barely knew anything about. The list of symptoms was long, but there was no way of knowing the severity of the issues our child would have, or what increased needs we would have to prepare for. However, the diagnosis would undoubtedly mean significant challenges and many adjustments.

John and I agreed to reach out to our family members on both sides to clarify any diseases or genetic abnormalities they may have had. I realized I didn't know why my mom's sister, Berit, had died at age seven. Kaori had other questions about our family histories we couldn't answer, so we promised to find out and get back to her. Before we left the office, we scheduled an appointment for the amniocentesis in a month. A month—it may as well be an eternity.

On our way home, we stopped and had lunch before we headed to the pharmacy to pick up the medicine for my nausea. It cost forty dollars for sixty pills. I was so tired of feeling nauseous that I didn't care how expensive the medication was. After the NIPT result, I felt both physically and emotionally exhausted.

We told our friends who already knew about the pregnancy about the potential issues and the need for further testing.

I never expected to be in this situation, but I guess that's the case for everyone. You always think, "It happens to others, but not me." Before Juni was born, I had been worried that I was too old when we decided to start a family, but my concern was only regarding fertility issues. I didn't think that there could be any issues once I was pregnant. I was wrong.

4

WORRY, WAITING, AND UNCERTAINTY

I didn't know what we would do if the fetus had a chromosomal abnormality. It's impossible to imagine this situation if you haven't experienced it. We didn't know if we would face a decision, but the risk was real, so we wanted to find as much information as possible.

I tended to be the more optimistic person in the family, but when we read about different scenarios, John embraced the potentially positive outcomes while I was fixated on the negative. I questioned why we would suddenly be "lucky." John believed we might be ready to take on the challenge of raising a child with a chromosomal abnormality, but I had my doubts. Those with children experiencing mild symptoms advocated for keeping the fetus, whereas those with severe symptoms argued against it. We would have to make up our minds with very little information. The coming weeks would be a brutal wait for answers.

Back at work, it wasn't easy to keep a poker face. Being cheerful was too much effort. I tried to avoid conversations about how I was doing. If anyone asked, I would tell them about my mom's surgery, and they would accept that as an explanation for my mood. I got nothing done beyond responding to emails.

Those who weren't aware of our situation may have thought I was behaving strangely, but I've always been an introverted person. Given my mom's situation, I didn't think anyone was suspicious. Even if they were, I didn't care. They weren't involved with what was going on in my life.

I felt guilty that I couldn't be a better mother. Juni didn't understand why her mom was crying all the time. She often kissed and hugged me and asked, "All good now, Mamma?"

I wished that all had been good.

I talked to my mom the day after her surgery. When I heard she was more alert, I couldn't pretend anymore.

"I'm so sorry to have to share this, especially now, but there is a risk that the fetus has a chromosome abnormality." I swallowed and couldn't stop the tears. "Can you please tell Dad, too? But please don't tell anyone else about the pregnancy or the test result, at least not yet."

"Oh, sweetheart, I wish I could hug you." I could feel her love through the phone. As a grandmother, she had agreed to wait for week 12 until telling family and friends that she was expecting a second grandchild. Now, her wait would be even longer.

"We've seen a genetic counselor, and she had some questions about our family. I know your sister Berit died, but what was the reason?"

"Yes, she died of scarlet fever when she was seven. But it all happened before I was born." I felt relieved that it wasn't because of a genetic condition.

After I had said goodbye to my mom, I called the genetic counselor. I left her a voicemail giving the answers my mom had provided. I missed her call a few hours later, so she left me a voicemail recommending another blood test. She said there was an increased risk that I had a gene mutation that could lead to spinal muscular atrophy (SMA) since my cousin has that genetic disorder. If both parents carry the gene mutation, it can cause SMA in the child. I would do the test first, and if I had the mutation, then John would too. She also mentioned that we could do the amniocentesis a few days sooner than we had scheduled. We wanted to do the blood test, but I hesitated to reschedule the amniocentesis. I knew getting it done as quickly as possible would be preferable, but parts of me wanted to stall. I didn't want to know. But if we were to terminate the pregnancy, it would be better to do it as soon as possible.

These were decisions I had hoped never to have to consider.

I took the next day off and couldn't fathom working the following week. There was no choice but to endure everything, one moment at a time. I tried to reach Kaori, but she didn't answer. I wrote a note on my calendar to call her again after the weekend. As if I could forget—I wasn't thinking of anything else.

When I reached Kaori, I told her we wanted to do the blood test and reschedule the amniocentesis. We didn't want to suffer through uncertainty any longer than necessary. The biggest question was what to do if the NIPT result was confirmed. We still didn't know.

John and I held on to hope that it was a false positive so we could forget this nightmare and move on without having to decide. But if the NIPT result was confirmed, what would we do? The doctors also suspected that the fetus had a heart defect, but they were unsure about the severity. Confirming the heart defect would require further tests, and they couldn't perform those until after the amniocentesis.

I never thought that we would find ourselves in a situation where we discussed an abortion. I had always thought a person had an abortion when you didn't want a child, not when you *wanted* a child. But we wanted a healthy child. We would love the child regardless, but would it be fair to give birth to a child who would have to live with challenges the rest of us would never have to consider? How long would the child live? And would it be fair to our daughter to be overshadowed by a younger sister who would require substantially more attention and help? The situation would be different if anyone in our family had been in an accident that affected their quality of life. But we could affect the outcome. Abortion was an option, but I knew that many people, especially here in the United States, would be critical of us for even considering ending the pregnancy.

But it was my body. It was my choice.

I texted my sister-in-law, Megan, wishing her a happy birthday. She responded that she sent "positive vibes to the baby." I broke down.

I understood why people say that you should refrain from telling anyone that you're pregnant until you've received confirmation that everything looks good, and you've reached at least week 12. Those who say, "Even if it's bad news, I'll share it anyway," don't know how it feels to receive disastrous news. Sure, if people had known about the pregnancy, they could've supported us, but we didn't want to discuss it before we decided what we wanted to do. I didn't even know how to describe my feelings and avoided talking to anyone but John.

On my day off, I drove to the Swedish Consulate to pick up my new passport. Some bad country song with lyrics about pain and sorrow that I didn't recognize was playing on the radio, and I felt my cheeks getting wet. The thought crossed my mind that I should continue driving away from everything as far as I could. But I knew it wouldn't solve my problems, just create new ones. Then, I thought that a car accident could be the solution—one where I survived without injuries but where the fetus didn't make it. Then I wouldn't have to decide. It would simply be a terrible accident. The thoughts were horrible. I had been considering seeing a therapist. Maybe I should do it sooner rather than later.

After the visit to the Consulate, I sat down to write about what had happened so far. I needed to process my thoughts and feelings somehow, and since I wasn't ready to talk about it, it had to be on paper. I felt so alone. It had all begun with what was supposed to be a routine test, but we had received unthinkable news.

Juni was at preschool, so I didn't have to pretend to feel well. Then I realized it was St. Patrick's Day, celebrated in memory of Ireland's patron saint, and the tradition in the United States is wearing green clothes. I suspected Juni was the only student not wearing shades of green because we hadn't realized the holiday was today. Hopefully she didn't care.

I wanted to forget my situation. In an attempt to escape reality, I read books and watched TV and movies, but there was always something to remind me. Parents who lost their children, life-changing doctor's appointments, people who tried to pretend everything was okay when it wasn't. I kept getting pulled back to my life.

I read Kristina Ohlsson's novel *The Flood*, where she writes about a character who goes through a similar experience. The woman gets annoyed when people think it would be good to know instead of worrying. But how can a diagnosis you don't want bring you peace? The only people who could think like that would be those who haven't experienced the same nightmare.

Her words hit too close to home. The uncertainty tortured me, but there was hope—not much, but better than if the amniocentesis confirmed the NIPT result, which would be my nightmare coming true. I wanted the torture of not knowing to end, but the problem was that it could become even worse.

Even though I could no longer bear reading more articles and posts on the internet, I still tormented myself. I knew more about chromosomal abnormalities than I ever wanted to know.

Before that fateful call from the doctor a few weeks earlier, we thought about whether the fetus would be a boy or a girl. We hoped child two would be a girl, but didn't dare say it out loud, because we would love a boy just as much. In retrospect, our previous thoughts felt naïve and pointless. Most expecting parents claim they don't care about the sex; they just want a healthy child. But if the child isn't healthy, what would they do then?

During our conversation, the doctor mentioned that the fetus in my womb was a girl, and again later, during the ultrasound, but I couldn't focus on it or enjoy it. All logic vanished, and I often caught myself thinking, *why wasn't it a boy? Maybe there wouldn't have been any problems then?* I felt like a terrible person and a terrible mother. It was a recurring feeling. I knew there wasn't anything John or I had done that had caused our situation. Sometimes, I still couldn't help but wonder if there was something we could have done differently.

John clung to the hope that the test result would be a false positive and hoped we would have a healthy girl. He looked forward to having another daughter and felt she would complete our family.

We had said before that we wouldn't discuss names until we knew the sex. Now, we decided we wouldn't discuss names until after we received the amniocentesis result. The genetic counselor had said it would take approximately ten days to get the result. If the news was good, they would call from the specialist clinic; if the news was bad, my doctor would likely call. I wished I would never see his number on my phone screen again.

We spent the weekend at home. I lacked energy and felt like

a zombie in the morning. I tried to turn off my thoughts and feelings by washing dishes and doing laundry, but it didn't work. John video-chatted with his parents and brothers, but I tried to avoid the screen. My mom called and told me she had received another blood transfusion and had a high fever. I broke down when I heard her exhausted voice. I couldn't respond when she went on to list relatives who had had genetic issues.

The doorbell rang after lunch, and we opened the door to see a box outside containing goodies and presents, including a soft yellow blanket that I immediately wrapped around myself. The box came with a card: *We heard that you have had some cloudy days, so here is a box of sunshine. Love Anne, Liz, and our families.* I valued my friendships so much, even though I couldn't handle spending time with any of my friends now.

John and Juni walked to the park. He tried to keep Juni busy to give me space to process everything. They did things together so she could keep a routine, even though I seldom felt well enough or had the energy to join them. John was also affected, of course, but not to the same degree. It was in my body that everything was happening. He thought a lot about our situation but could compartmentalize that part of his life when necessary. He had left the TV on, and by chance, I watched the end of a March Madness basketball game between the favored team, Villanova, and the lower-ranked team, Wisconsin. I couldn't help but think of the parallel. Like Wisconsin, we also hoped for a miracle. Unfortunately, fate wasn't in our hands, and I could use a timeout. To my delight, Wisconsin won the game. We still had several weeks before we would know how our "game" would end.

During Juni's birth, the doctor thought for a moment that I would need an emergency cesarean section. Juni's heartbeat was too slow, and nothing the doctors and nurses tried helped.

They rolled me into the operating room, gave me anesthesia, and prepared me for surgery. I'll never forget the feeling I had during those minutes. I didn't know where John was or if our daughter would survive. But then, thankfully, her heart rate increased. They rolled me back to the delivery room, where John waited with scrubs on. I ended up having a vaginal delivery. But that dreadful feeling of worry and uncertainty had returned and was constant. The fear and uncertainty had been with me for weeks now.

My feelings were a rollercoaster. I felt down and helpless, but every so often, I found solace in the hope of a false positive. My internet searches continued, and I embraced the stories about women who had gone through similar experiences and received a false positive. I knew it might not end like that for us, but to get through the next month, I needed to think about it, at least sometimes.

It was Wednesday, and the rain was pouring down. It suited my mood better than the sunny weather typical of Southern California. I talked to my mom early in the morning, and she said she might get discharged from the hospital the following day. It was later than they first had estimated, but it was a relief that things were going in the right direction.

I talked to my friend Anne later in the day. She and her husband, Jason, had a scary experience during the first ultrasound of their first child. The doctor saw some white spots on the brain of the fetus and suspected trisomy 13. Four weeks later, another ultrasound showed that it was incorrect. But those weeks were torture for them. We were experiencing the same torture now. I tried to cling to hope. My doctor told me he only had one other patient with the same test result as us during all his years practicing medicine. Her amniocentesis confirmed the diagnosis.

I hoped that our result would be different.

World Down Syndrome Day is on March 21. In Sweden, people "rocked the socks"—wearing mismatched socks to show that they celebrate differences. The debate raged in online forums and blogs, where many believed it was a double standard to rock your socks and still do prenatal testing. I read and cried. Likely, those critics had never been in my shoes. It's far too easy to be opinionated about things you haven't experienced.

I read this on Twitter: "Remember sitting in history, thinking 'If I was alive then, I would've...' You're alive now. Whatever you're doing is what you would've done." You may fool yourself, but your current behavior reflects how you would have acted in the past. It's easy to talk or think, but what actions would you take when it really matters?

In the 2017 season, the first episode of the Swedish documentary TV series *The Correspondents* covered the abortion issue in Poland, Norway, and the United States. An American woman shared her experience of having an abortion for medical reasons. She already had two biological daughters and was also a foster mom to other children with special needs. Yet people were standing outside the abortion clinic and screaming at her, saying she was a horrible human being. Talking is simple; acting isn't. If only the protesters had more compassion, they could have used their time and energy to help others instead.

A few days later, I received an email from my mom with the message, *Home again!* Finally, some good news, but we were still waiting for her test results. In other news from Sweden we found out that Princess Sofia and Prince Carl Philip were expecting their second child in September. I wondered if we would have a baby then, too. I read how Princess Sofia and the fetus were healthy and doing well, and the envy burned in me. All I wanted was a healthy baby. I didn't believe in God, but I prayed to all higher powers I could think of. I feared that my negative thoughts might harm the fetus, but I couldn't help it. I couldn't stop.

I declined a coworker's baby shower invitation, saying I wasn't feeling well. I felt guilty for not celebrating with her, but I wasn't in the mood to be surrounded by cheerful exclamations when guests see the baby clothes. That same night, John's brother James came over for dinner. He was in town for business, and luckily, his work paid for his hotel, so he didn't ask if he could stay with us. I couldn't bear to hang out with anyone, no matter who it was.

My tears were a constant presence as the days went on. I cried on the inside all the time. John and I worked from home, so we often ate lunch together, giving us time to talk undisturbed. There were countless tears, and my feelings overpowered me at one lunch. Amid my tears, John listened and provided support.

"You know I love you, and I'll never judge you, no matter what we decide to do, right?" he asked, but it wasn't a question.

I believed him. The problem was I might judge myself.

I hoped, more than anything I had hoped for in a long time, that we wouldn't have to decide. Then, no one would need to find out what we had planned on doing if the diagnosis was confirmed. After all our research and our discussions, I was pretty sure I wanted to have an abortion if the NIPT result was confirmed, but I couldn't know for sure until then. It was impossible to know how I would feel if we had to face a decision. Ultimately, I wanted the best for our family, daughter, and future child.

Not everyone gets the opportunity to decide. Many families don't receive a diagnosis until after the birth of their child. Even though it's taboo to talk about, some wish they could have made an informed decision with the family's best interest in mind.

I grieved every day. I grieved for something I imagined. I grieved every day that I couldn't be happy for the family I already had. I grieved every day that I had already lost.

Sara and Eddie came over for dinner and to watch basketball. March Madness was still going on. They brought pizza, which we were grateful for since we didn't want to cook. I still didn't feel like hanging out with anyone. I curled up in the couch's corner, but the rest of my family was happy to have company. The game lasted past Juni's bedtime, but she got to watch her tablet and was content. Jealousy stormed inside me when John and Eddie wanted to go to the bar across the street for a beer after the game. My entire world was in turmoil, and there was nothing I could do to escape, but they could leave, have a beer, and relax. I understood John wanted a break from everything, but it felt unfair. The fetus was growing inside of me, and I carried it with me everywhere. I wished I could have taken a break from my body.

I talked to Sara again the following day. Her due date was two months away. She and Eddie had just attended a birthing class, and she had a lot of questions about the birthing plan, the birth itself, and newborns.

"You don't care what happens as long as the baby is healthy," she said. There it was again, that haunting sentiment. I swallowed. I don't think she realized how this statement affected me. How many times haven't you heard the same thing being said? I didn't know what to say. I considered my possible outcomes: either I would have a miscarriage, I would birth a healthy child, or we would face a confirmed chromosomal abnormality diagnosis, and then we would have to decide whether to have an abortion. I barely said anything before we ended the call. I didn't want my negativity to ruin their happiness.

It was hardly a surprise that I was angry and disappointed when Donald Trump was elected president. We knew that he and other Republicans would try to pass healthcare cuts. What I didn't realize was how it would affect me on such a personal and emotional level. If their bills passed, then healthcare for women wouldn't only become more expensive but disappear in many places around the country. It's shocking and sad how ruthless people can be.

The bill wouldn't only affect women but also individuals lacking jobs, money, or health insurance. In his talk show, comedian and talk show host Jimmy Kimmel talked about the heart defect his newborn son Billy had been born with. He criticized Donald Trump and said, "If your baby is going to die but it doesn't have to, it shouldn't matter how much money you make."

We were relieved when Donald Trump and the Republican party withdrew the first of their healthcare reform bills. But they would continue to try passing other bills, each one worse than the other.

Healthcare discussions were everywhere. I couldn't escape discussions about women's right to healthcare and women's rights to their bodily autonomy. On TV, at work, on social media, at home, in my own body—I couldn't escape no matter what. All I could do was continue to wait.

5

ABORTION RIGHTS IN THE UNITED STATES

Views on abortion are very different in the United States compared to Sweden, and the right to abortion is a constant topic in American political debates. It's one of the most controversial issues in American politics and culture.

With a republican president in power, abortion rights faced renewed scrutiny and attack. Republicans introduced several bills attempting to limit abortion rights throughout Trump's first year as president. Since we were considering abortion, it was extra painful that so many Americans didn't think we should have that right. Seven out of ten Americans supported the right to abortion, but there was still a loud segment that didn't.

When the United States became independent in 1776, abortion was legal in most states until you could feel fetal movement. In the late 1800s, all states passed different anti-abortion laws. The reason wasn't religion or politics then, but because the medications taken to induce abortions posed a poisoning risk. At least, that was the explanation given. During this time, women had ambitions outside the home, and the anti-abortion movement opposed these ambitions. There was also a racist agenda since abortions and contraceptives were leading to a decreasing number of births among white women at the same time as immigration was increasing. This trend frightened people who wanted whites to remain the majority.

Abortion and contraceptives returned to the spotlight when the women's rights movement gained momentum in the 1960s, since they are fundamental aspects of equality and the fight for women's rights. Today, religion and morality are the principal arguments against abortion. However, restricting access to safe and legal abortions is a way to control women. It's sadly as true today as it was one hundred years ago.

The Supreme Court's landmark decision in *Roe v. Wade* was a crucial step forward for abortion rights in the United States. But despite being legal across the nation since 1973, abortion is still, sadly, not regarded as a standard healthcare procedure in the United States.

The Supreme Court overturned *Roe v. Wade* after I submitted my manuscript to my Swedish publisher.

In 1969, when Norma McCorvey was twenty-two years old, she wanted an abortion. But she couldn't get one since abortion was illegal in Texas unless her life was at risk. Similar laws existed in most other states. McCorvey sued Henry Wade, the District Attorney of Dallas County, using the pseudonym Jane Roe. She appealed the case to the Supreme Court, which ruled that a woman may make her own medical decisions, including the decision to have an abortion. The verdict made abortion legal nationwide in the United States.

The ruling happened over forty-five years ago, so why is the number of abortion clinics decreasing? Access to contraceptives could be a reason, which some Republicans also want to limit. Some states, like Kentucky, only have one abortion clinic, and opponents hope even that will close. Fewer abortion clinics result in increased expenses, causing delays in obtaining abortions. Travel, lodging, and abortion expenses can be out of reach for many. A second-trimester abortion in 2017 could cost as much as $3,000, and some health insurance policies don't cover abortion costs. Copays differ, and some people lack health insurance coverage entirely. Saving up the money and organizing transportation takes time, further delaying abortions.

In some states, you must travel over 170 miles to get to an abortion clinic. This makes it even more difficult logistically and financially since many states have laws requiring women to wait eighteen to seventy-two hours after counseling before they can go through with the abortion. It's not only the stigma against abortions that makes it difficult—restrictive laws and financial constraints also play a significant role.

Violence against abortion providers and abortion clinics is a part of life in the United States. Arsons and death threats are far too common. Someone shot and killed Doctor George Tiller, a famous abortion provider, while he was attending church on May 31, 2009, and there was no doubt about the motive. The killer was against abortion. Bill O'Reilly had spoken critically about Dr. Tiller several times on his TV show. A tragic mass shooting at a Planned Parenthood clinic in Colorado Springs in November 2015 claimed the lives of three people and left nine injured. Abortion opponents often publish abortion providers' names, addresses, and phone numbers on different websites. The threats and violence explain why the clinics need bulletproof glass.

Some healthcare providers are transparent, but others choose not to advertise what they do. I read about an abortion provider, Dr. Krajewski, whose personal relationships often have ended, sometimes before they even started, because of her career. She had a coat hanger, the symbol for illegal abortions, tattooed on her arm. She said: "Whatever happens, I will no longer be silent or fearful when a new love interest—or anyone —makes me feel exposed and vulnerable. As my tattoo says: Never again." I admire her strength and courage.

The abortion issue is very polarizing in the United States. Some support safe and legal abortions; this is often called the "pro-choice" stance. Others oppose safe and legal abortions, which is often called the "pro-life" stance. The language we use matters. The same people who say they are pro-life often also support the death penalty and don't want to limit access to guns in efforts to reduce gun violence. And many aren't interested in supporting programs that assist new mothers after their baby is born. This group's successful adoption of the term "pro-life" has benefited their interests despite their conflicting views on the sanctity of life in other areas. We all have a responsibility to highlight the misinformation and stigma that contributes to a culture where anti-abortion support grows, especially as it becomes easier to enact laws that limit access.

The distinction made between "good" and "bad" abortions is also problematic. When people say that abortions should only be legal if the woman's life is in danger or in cases of rape, we are treading on thin ice. These debates reinforce the view that some abortions are acceptable, but not all, which still opposes the right for women's full autonomy over their bodies. Abortion is a personal decision, and no one should have to defend or explain themselves. Ultimately, the decision should lie with the pregnant woman.

The conservative Christian right, known for their immense political influence, plays a crucial role in the anti-abortion movement. It's mind-boggling how religion takes precedence over scientific evidence and logic. Facts are irrelevant to them. President Trump shares their attitude, and they support him.

Some right-wing evangelical Christians are considered hate

groups because of their extreme beliefs. Some even back the death penalty for those who have an abortion. While there may be exceptions, the Democratic party supports safe and legal abortions, while most Republicans oppose them. My political party affiliation is obvious.

In the United States, Planned Parenthood is a leading advocate for safe and legal abortions. This nonprofit health organization has been serving the community for over one hundred years. Planned Parenthood runs over six hundred health centers across all fifty states and Washington, DC. They are funded by federal funds, private insurance, fees, and donations. Their services range from sexual education and contraceptives to STI tests, treatments, cancer screenings, and, in some clinics, abortions. One in every five women in the United States has visited Planned Parenthood.

In 1916, the first birth control clinic opened in Brooklyn, New York, marking the beginning of the organization's history. At that time contraceptives and abortions were illegal. By the late 1960s, the number of clinics in the United States had surpassed four hundred, and people mostly disregarded the contraceptive ban. The state of New York legalized abortion in 1970, and the Planned Parenthood clinic in Syracuse was the first to offer abortions. Abortion became available in more clinics when *Roe v. Wade* made abortion legal in the entire country.

Even though abortions are legal in all states, access varies because the American healthcare system doesn't mandate hospitals and medical groups to provide abortion services. Before I moved to the United States, I didn't know how the American healthcare system worked. Today I work for a medical group, but I still struggle to comprehend how it's structured.

Sweden has long had universal health coverage, primarily

funded by tax revenue. Covered services range from inpatient and outpatient care to dental, mental health, long-term care, and prescription drugs. Some services require copayments, but there is an annual maximum limit on how much you pay. Some groups, like children and older people, aren't required to pay. All residents have the same rights to receive care, with priority given to those in greatest need. Some Democrats want a system more like Sweden's, but I'm skeptical about its feasibility in the United States.

Today, Planned Parenthood is the largest individual organization that offer abortions in the United States. In many places, they are the only healthcare organization to do so. However, it's important to note that they would perform fewer abortions if doctors would perform abortions themselves instead of referring their patients to Planned Parenthood.

Even though abortions only make up a small portion of their services, Planned Parenthood has become synonymous with everything that abortion opponents despise; they have even made false claims about Planned Parenthood selling fetal tissue. Republicans have proposed bills that target Planned Parenthood in an effort to cut federal funding unless they stop performing abortions. Making it harder for women to have safe and legal abortions is the initial step toward their goal of eliminating abortion access entirely. But ending all funding for Planned Parenthood would have massive repercussions, given its crucial role in the American healthcare system. So far, the abortion opponents have failed, and Planned Parenthood marked its one hundredth anniversary in 2017.

The year 2017 brought major setbacks for abortion rights in the United States. In nineteen states, 63 new bills were passed to restrict abortion rights and availability. Between 2011 and 2017, states passed 401 restrictions. Many of these bills are in direct conflict with scientific evidence, but the politicians behind them don't seem to care. Women become the victims.

States can implement restrictions if not challenged in court or vetoed by governors. State restrictions on abortion include gestational limits, mandatory counseling, waiting periods, mandatory ultrasounds, physician licensing requirements, clinic building codes, and parental consent for minors. The list is endless. There's a law in Texas that prevents patients from suing doctors who withhold prenatal test results. Caregivers may deceive their patients under this law to prevent abortions. Democratic governors in some states prevented the passing of new restrictive laws by using their veto power.

The states pushing for radical restrictions ultimately wanted the Supreme Court to revisit the abortion case and overturn *Roe v. Wade*—a frightening possibility given the conservative majority on the court.

In 2017, only 30 percent of women in the United States lived in a state that was supportive of abortion rights. California was one of those states. The other eleven states were Washington, Oregon, Montana, New Mexico, Maine, Vermont, Connecticut, New York, New Jersey, Maryland, and Hawaii.

I always answer without hesitation when relatives ask if we would ever consider moving to another state. I couldn't move to a state that is hostile to abortion rights, not just for me but for Juni's sake. Even though I hope she'll never need an abortion, I want her to have the option.

6

ALL IS NOT WELL

It was Monday morning, and I sat at the desk in my home office. While my work computer was starting up, I checked Facebook on my phone. I saw a post by my husband's aunt: "It's been one year ago today that I said goodbye to my mother. I hope she is now at peace with my father. Just in case they don't know, we are expecting 2 new babies this year and all is well." It ended with a heart emoji.

I was grateful Juni got to meet John's grandmother while she was still alive, but John's aunt wasn't supposed to know I was pregnant. I knew her grandchild's wife was pregnant, but I didn't know who she meant in the family if she wasn't talking about us. It had to have been us.

I hurried upstairs to John and collapsed on the floor. My voice broke, and it took a while before I could get the words out to explain why I was so upset. He promised to talk to his mom. She had promised not to say anything, but had she done it anyway? John suspected as much but didn't want me to be mad at her. But if that Facebook post was about us, all was not well —far from it.

John's mom had told his aunt. My heart raced. The aunt removed the last sentence in the post after John spoke with his mom, but I was still angry and disappointed. I didn't want the news to spread. A close colleague who knew about my pregnancy had told her boss, but she told me right away. I appreciated that, so it didn't catch me off guard when the boss saw me in the office lobby, where she asked how I was feeling and why I hadn't shared the pregnancy news. I sighed and thought, *You shouldn't even know*.

It hurt that my mother-in-law shared the news without giving us a heads-up. Also, there wasn't a baby yet, only a fetus.

I stayed home when John, Juni, and John's brother, James, went to the park a few days later. The doorbell rang, and a flower delivery person stood outside the door. I assumed they were from a friend, but when I opened the card, it said: *I am sorry. Aunt P.* I texted her, saying that I accepted her apology and thanked her for the beautiful bouquet. We didn't know how much she knew, but I didn't want to go into details.

If the result of the amniocentesis confirmed a false positive, we would have another daughter in September. If not, I didn't know if I would be pregnant this summer. I felt like a terrible person. The flowers reminded me that more people than I wanted knew I was pregnant. I didn't dare to think about the consequences of a terminated pregnancy. What would people think and say then? James came over for dinner, saw the bouquet, and asked who it was from. When I told him, he shook his head, sighed, and said, "I'm not surprised."

Following the genetic counselor's advice, we went to the laboratory closest to our house for the recommended blood test due to the SMA gene in my family. I bumped into people I knew from work and said everything was going great when they asked how I was doing. I whispered a *thank you* when the lab staff didn't say the test name out loud when they called my name. The discretion felt respectful.

I browsed Swedish internet bookstores searching for books relevant to our situation. I didn't know what category to choose: family, health, parenting, pregnancy, or disease management. No matter what terms I used, I couldn't find any results. Why were there no books on this subject? Was there no one who wanted to share their experiences? Feeling alone, I would have found comfort in reading about someone in a similar position. If people were more open about their experiences, it would be harder to stigmatize abortion.

As the first trimester ended, I felt *very* pregnant, which made me very uncomfortable. I looked pregnant, too, if I wore tight clothes. My first and second pregnancies were noticeably different. It seemed like my body remembered and stretched out quicker this time. I tried to hide my pregnancy and keep it from everyone, even though the constant nausea made it impossible to forget. I would have preferred to wear normal or maternity clothes, but I hid beneath yoga pants and baggy college sweaters. I felt ugly, sick, and dull; the entire year had been one long agony.

The sun was shining, and the sky was blue, so we went on a short walk. Torrential rain and thunderstorms would have suited my mood better. My discomfort had gone so far that even the weather annoyed me.

My mom had more doctors' appointments lined up, where they would examine different parts of her body they hadn't already checked. She was at home resting after the surgery, and she was worried about what the future would bring—the same status as mine.

As the end of March drew near, we could do the amniocentesis soon. Time had passed so slowly, but the test was only done between the fifteenth and twentieth week of pregnancy. Then, the analysis would take two to three weeks to complete.

In a month we would know the test result. In about two months, I would either have an enormous belly and hopefully no nausea, or I wouldn't be pregnant anymore, and I couldn't handle that thought.

John and his brother James went out with two friends on Friday night, and I couldn't help but feel jealous. He could leave the situation and enjoy a social life. That wasn't an option for me. The only thing ahead of me was another sleepless night.

Every year, I would attend a conference on women's health. The event aimed to inspire women to live a healthier and more balanced life. In breakout sessions, inspirational speakers from different fields gave lectures on health and lifestyle topics. In the main ballroom, you could get pampered with a massage or manicure and get free health screenings. I debated attending this year's event because I was still feeling nauseous, uncomfortable, and anxious. But since Sara was going, I decided to join her. If it got too overwhelming, I could leave the conference early.

We attended some lectures after breakfast. The first was called Reducing Emotional Suffering: How to Ride Life's Highs and Lows. It was an appropriate topic. The speaker, a psychologist, explained how to differentiate between sadness and depression. She presented a checklist, and it didn't surprise me when I could check several boxes on the list of signs leading to depression. Her advice was to talk or write about your feelings and experiences.

We attended another captivating lecture in the afternoon: *The Choice: Escape the Past and Embrace the Possible*. The speaker, author, and psychologist Dr. Edith Eva Eger was sent to the Auschwitz concentration camp with her family when she was sixteen. She and her sister were the sole survivors of their family. She said forgiveness freed her from her mental prison. Now, Dr. Eger helps her patients cope with trauma, grief, and abuse. Her response was commendable; she couldn't control her circumstances but controlled her reaction. While her experiences were unspeakably cruel compared to mine, I still didn't know how to confront the seemingly impossible decision if it came to that.

Back at work, I struggled to focus. While working on a report on one computer screen, I opened the search engine on another. I saw Camilla Gervide's "Better Place (Tille's Song)" and pressed play. Camilla wrote the song for Tille, a young Swedish boy who died because of the disease Epidermolysis bullosa. The lyrics, describing how heaven lost an angel and sent for him, hit me in the heart. She tells how he's in a better place where there's no sorrow or pain, and he'll never be far away as he shines in every star she sees. My tears flowed as I listened. I didn't know how things would end, but I was in pain.

My eyes grew puffier and puffier as I continued playing sad songs on repeat. I was supposed to work, but my emotions overwhelmed me. I grieved for a daughter I may never have the chance to know. That Juni may never have a sibling, a sister, filled me with sorrow. As I reached for the nearest tissue package, I saw it came from the gift bag from Saturday's conference, sponsored by the Hospital for Women and Newborns. My gut twisted. The workday ended as the last notes of Laleh's "Some Die Young" played. I turned off the computer, my cheeks still wet.

I was thinking a lot about the differences between Sweden and the United States. I had lived in the United States since the late 1990s, for most of my adult life. When I first moved abroad, I didn't consider the impact it would have on my life. I felt a sense of belonging in both countries' cultures and daily life. However, I had to admit that I had only lived on the American coasts, first a year on the East Coast and on the West Coast since then.

I have had little personal experience with "middle America" or the states between the Atlantic and Pacific coasts. I visited some of these states while working for a company that catered to coal companies. Although I wasn't proud of working there, I had to pay rent, and they agreed to sponsor my work visa, so I took the job. Despite my guilt over supporting coal companies, I tried to be a good person in other aspects of my life. Sometimes, we would visit John's relatives in Kentucky, Tennessee, Missouri, and Georgia. I had a feeling that some of them might oppose the right to safe and legal abortion, but I didn't know; it was never a topic of conversation.

When John's cousin Susan was getting married in 2012, I attended a wedding luncheon in Nashville, Tennessee. We sat at round tables, talking as we waited for the food.

"You know he's married to a foreigner, right?" a woman at my table said about one of the bride's brothers.

"He couldn't find an American woman that would marry him?" The woman beside her chuckled, jumping at the chance to gossip.

Simona, who was married to another brother of the bride, was Italian and seated at our table. Their comments left us both speechless. They hadn't realized we were immigrants.

"I'm from Sweden, and she's from Italy," I said, gesturing toward Simona, unsure where this would take their conversation.

My words caught them off guard, but to remedy the situation, one of them said, "Well, I can't tell that you're not American. Europe is different, and I've been to Sweden; it was lovely."

I didn't know what to say. Fortunately, the servers intervened by placing lunch plates in front of us, diverting my attention to the meal. This luncheon took place long before Donald Trump became president.

April 7, 2017, started with the shocking news of a terrorist attack in Stockholm, Sweden. I spoke to my sister, and she knew where all our family members in Stockholm were except for our nephew. I turned on the Swedish TV channel and followed the news in shock, hoping our nephew was safe. After a few minutes, my sister called to let me know she had found out where our nephew was. Everyone in my family was unharmed. I let out a sigh of relief.

I reached out to my parents, who were unaware of the attack as they had been at the hospital all day. The doctors had confirmed that my mother had lymphoma, cancer of the lymphatic system. They were uncertain about the type, so she needed further tests. With the Swedish news on in the background, I worked in a state of shock. Everything seemed to be falling apart.

The hashtag #openstockholm quickly started trending on social media as people in Stockholm offered their homes and help to those affected. Amid all the horror, there was still hope. My emotions were on a rollercoaster that weekend. I felt gratitude and pride for being Swedish, but I also ached to be in Sweden and desperately missed my family.

A few days after the terrorist attack, I read in Swedish newspapers about a midwife who sued her home region when they didn't employ her because she refused to perform abortions, insert IUDs, or distribute morning-after pills. She lost the case. She had no grounds for claiming discrimination when her job application as a midwife was rejected, and she couldn't challenge the decision. Once again, I was proud of Sweden.

John and I rewatched the TV series *Friends* to escape reality as we waited for the amniocentesis. We were watching the episodes where Monica and Chandler were going to adopt a child. In one of them, the mother of the child they were going to adopt didn't know who the biological father of the child was —her high school boyfriend, who was an American football player, or a man who had killed his father with a shovel. As I thought about our upcoming test and the result, I couldn't help but feel like Chandler when he said, "Honey, it's us. Of course it's the shovel killer."

7

THE AMNIOCENTESIS

E arly Monday morning, I woke up with a knot in my stomach. It was that same feeling you get before holding a presentation or going on a first date, but this wasn't for a pleasant or exciting reason. We left around 9:00 a.m., and when we arrived at the specialist's office, I had to go to the bathroom several times before they finally called my name. First, they performed an ultrasound that lasted about forty minutes. They showed us the fetus, and we watched it move while they completed the measurements and examinations.

In some American states, laws require a doctor to describe and show the images from the ultrasound to the pregnant woman and force her to listen to the fetus's heartbeat before she can have an abortion in attempts to tug on heartstrings and dissuade them from going through with it. I suffer with the women of these states. There is no reason to be forced into this when you have already made your decision.

The doctor and nurse commented on how active the fetus was, bringing back memories of my pregnancy with Juni. She would constantly wiggle and do somersaults. It seemed like this fetus had a similar personality. I couldn't bring myself to look when the test began. The procedure was uncomfortable but not as painful as I had expected. They took two test tubes containing pale yellow fluid but assured me that there was enough left for the fetus. We received pictures from the ultrasound, and I put them in my purse without looking at them. They told us to expect results in eight to ten days, maybe even longer.

I got up, but everything was spinning, so I had to grab on to John. The doctor requested that I return in four weeks for an echocardiogram to examine the fetus's heart further. We scheduled the appointment before heading to the elevator that took us to the parking garage. They told me to rest and minimize physical movement for the next twenty-four hours, so I parked myself on the couch when we got home.

John picked up Juni from preschool in the afternoon. I heard the garage door open and her little feet coming up the stairs. Her face lit up with a smile when she saw me, and she ran up to hug me.

"Hi, sweetie, I love you." I hugged her back but had to stop her from crawling onto my lap.

"But Mamma, why?" It was difficult to explain why she couldn't sit on my lap. It made no sense to her. John had to come and grab her. After a snack, she climbed onto the couch and snuggled next to me. We both needed the closeness. I had cramps, and I kept telling myself it was normal, but I took two days off just in case.

Back at work on Thursday, I continued to battle with persistent nausea and anxiety. We were back to waiting again. It felt like waiting periods defined my whole life.

The following day, I was supposed to be in the office for an all-day audit, but with everything going on, I was too distracted. I took another day off; fortunately, others in our department could cover for me.

I spent the weekend on the couch reading *The Girl Before* by JP Delaney. As usual, I couldn't escape my situation, but I felt a glimmer of hope when I read the sentence: "After all, the odds are still vastly in favor of everything being fine. Thousands of expectant mothers have a scare like this, only to discover that's all it ever was: a scare."

8

THE TEST RESULT

Seven days had passed since the amniocentesis. According to the specialist, it could take anywhere from eight to ten days, or maybe even longer, to get the results. We were incredibly nervous. For some reason, I thought that the longer the wait, the more likely the news would be negative. My thoughts made no sense, but my emotions trumped logic. Desperate, I prayed to higher powers that the fetus would be healthy because I couldn't bear the alternative.

My phone chimed with a notification, and I saw my mom had emailed me. *Hi, I saw the hematologist today. There's nothing to medicate now. The bone marrow was also good. The ureter they removed earlier contained lymphoma, but they found no more. But it may come back later, in a few years, or not at all. They'll monitor me, so I'll go back for tests in 3 months, and they'll check to see if I'm well. The polyp that started it all has nothing to do with this, so the gynecologist will also keep an eye on me. Kisses and hugs.*

This news brought me relief and happiness. If only the good news could keep coming.

Later that day, I had a meeting at the office, so I rummaged through my closet, looking for clothes to cover up the pregnancy. I decided on a black suit with a loose-fitting shirt. John advised me to keep the jacket open because if I buttoned it, my pregnancy showed. I let my long hair hang loose, hiding my enlarged breasts. Only two of my colleagues knew I was pregnant. I went to the office and held my stomach in as best I could. We hadn't told Juni that I was pregnant yet. Whenever she pointed out that my stomach looked different, I told her I had a burrito in my tummy, which wasn't unlikely since Mexican food was a family favorite.

When I arrived home, I changed into yoga pants and let out a deep exhale. As soon as I sat down in my office chair, my cell phone started ringing. Seeing Kaori's number on the caller ID brought me hope. It had only been eight days since the test. Hadn't she said the doctor would call if there was bad news? I took a deep breath before I pressed the button to answer.

Within minutes, my world fell apart.

The test had confirmed the suspicions from the NIPT test, and the chromosomal abnormality was now a diagnosis. It was impossible to anticipate the full extent of the impact on the child before birth. Still, it was certain there would be increased needs. Frequent visits to speech therapists, physiotherapists, and specialist doctors would become routine. She continued talking about the heart defect and additional tests, but all I could hear was my own heart pounding.

We hung up, and something inside me broke. I knew it would never fully heal. I struggled to catch my breath, pressure weighing on my chest, and the tears were impossible to stop. I was drowning in feelings I had never felt before. My legs were heavy as I walked upstairs to our bedroom and collapsed on the floor. I couldn't get out what Kaori had said, but John understood. I was utterly devastated. All energy had been sucked out of my body. I never knew that it could hurt so much. We knew this was possible, but preparing for what it would feel like was impossible. We had kept hoping for a different outcome; now, our hope was crushed.

John contacted the genetic counselor and scheduled an appointment for the following day. We postponed the final decision until then. Dr. Robertson had suggested that we see Kaori again, and we felt obliged to follow his advice.

When I informed my manager that I needed time off, she understood and assured me it wasn't an issue. Tears continued to fall as the afternoon and evening drifted by in a haze. Juni couldn't understand why her hugs couldn't make me happy again—my little girl who may never become a big sister.

9

THE DECISION

I had trouble sleeping, and I feared what would happen. I showered and put on a pair of maternity pants. They were the only clothes that fit. We went to the genetic counselor's office. After a while in the waiting room, we were ushered into the small, windowless room that served as Kaori's office. She had nothing to say that we didn't already know. No one could tell us how severely the child would be affected by the chromosomal abnormality, but we knew that it would alter our lives. It would affect us as parents; Juni's life would change, and the child would face unique challenges that the rest of us didn't have to consider. The fetus also had a suspected heart defect, but a diagnosis required further testing. Kaori couldn't provide any indication of how severe that defect was, either. There were so many unknowns.

We had read all the articles we could find about the chromosomal abnormality. We talked about what others in the same situation tended to do. John pressured Kaori to provide statistics. We wanted to know how common the chromosomal abnormality was and how often people in the same situation chose abortion. She had no answers.

We also discussed the risk of a similar thing happening in a future pregnancy. Kaori clarified that the diagnosis wasn't hereditary. It was because of a random event when the cells formed. Therefore, the risk of the same diagnosis was minimal. But given my age, there were increased risks overall. Tears welled up as I considered the possibility of reliving a similar experience. We asked a few more questions before we headed home.

We sat next to each other on the couch, John squeezing my hand. There was a long moment of silence. And then I said it.

"I want us to have an abortion."

John nodded in agreement and said without hesitation, "I want the same thing." He would have agreed with me no matter what I had said because he knew it was ultimately up to me and accepted what I wanted, but it felt like a mutual decision. Choosing to have an abortion and end the pregnancy was the best decision for our family. It felt surreal that it was official.

Our focus shifted to getting the abortion scheduled. I called the medical group, and they assured me my doctor would call back the same day. We tried to distract ourselves while waiting for his call by watching movies. It didn't work. I couldn't stop thinking about it. Soon, I would be one of many women who have had an abortion.

I called my mom and told her. She felt sorry for us but believed we had made the right decision. I messaged the friends I had shared the pregnancy news with, and they responded with kindness and understanding. A friend told me that several of her friends had had abortions. I appreciated their supportive responses.

John had a job interview in the afternoon, so I drove to pick up Juni from preschool. It had been so long since I was there that I didn't remember the gate code, so I had to text my friend Liz, whose daughter attended the same preschool. Juni's reaction to seeing me was pure delight, and I tried my best to hold my stomach in to prevent unwanted questions. We returned home, and John and Juni walked to the library after his interview.

When they got home just after six, the phone rang again.

"Hello, this is Dr. Robertson. Sorry it took me a while to get back to you, and I'm so sorry about the result." I took a breath.

"Yes, we're devastated, and we've decided to have an abortion." There, I said it out loud to someone other than John.

"I get it, and if it makes you feel any better, I would have done the same thing. My wife did amniocenteses for all her pregnancies when she was thirty-two, thirty-six, and thirty-nine." It didn't help me feel better, but at least I didn't feel judged.

"It's crazy how it's so different here compared to Sweden. I wish having an abortion wasn't such a big deal. It should just be healthcare, not politics." I reached for a tissue.

"Yes, it's very different here, unfortunately." He explained what would happen next. The procedure—I couldn't even say the word "abortion" and realized that I, too, was a victim of society's taboo—would take two days, so, unfortunately, it couldn't happen until next week. Two days? My head was spinning. Why had no one told me it would take two days?

"I'll call the insurance company and Planned Parenthood after this. It's better if they do the abortion. They're experts, and I want you to get the best care possible. But I'll help you make all the arrangements." I was surprised he sent me away, but I was so overwhelmed by the situation that I didn't question it. It irritated John when I told him because Dr. Robertson had implied during our appointment that he would perform the procedure if we elected to have an abortion. But because of the intense political controversy surrounding abortion, John assumed that was the explanation and left it at that.

"Have you thought about whether you'll try to conceive again?" Dr. Robertson asked.

"It's too early to think about that," I answered. We had hesitated about two children, so perhaps our family was already complete. Only the future could tell.

"Well, you take care now, and I promise I'll call you tomorrow," he said, and we ended the call. I felt grateful to have such a compassionate and understanding doctor. It made a difficult thing—the hardest thing I had ever done—just a little easier.

I had a sleepless night. In the morning, I called and canceled all upcoming doctors' appointments, including the routine ultrasound scheduled for week 18 and the specialist visit in three weeks. When they asked why, the tears came before I could even answer.

I spent most of the day doing laundry, cleaning, and organizing things. John took apart the changing table we had kept even though Juni had stopped wearing diapers, and something inside of me shattered even more. The future we had imagined looked completely different now. Instead of two children, we would have only one. I didn't dare consider another pregnancy yet.

John respected my feelings and supported me in my grief. It was more tangible to me because it was happening in my body, but John was also sad and upset that this was happening to us. For him to tackle the changing table project so quickly was a rare initiative on his part. He normally procrastinated on household projects until I reminded him multiple times. He said he got an outlet for his grief by doing something practical.

My mom called, and she had told my dad. He was sad but acknowledged our strength in making this decision. John called his parents to let them know. The conversations were emotional. Painful.

Dr. Robertson contacted me to let me know he had sent the

information to the insurance company. After we ended our conversation, I called Planned Parenthood to schedule the appointment. They still needed my medical records before I could make an appointment. It would probably be Tuesday and Wednesday the following week—more waiting.

The following day, Planned Parenthood called me several times. They had received my medical records but still needed to verify that the paperwork was in order. They also needed more information about my health insurance. Once everything was sorted out, and after a bit of phone tag, I got an appointment scheduled for Tuesday. It was going to be a long weekend.

The Swedish Consulate and Swedish Chamber of Commerce organized an event on the beach to celebrate the Swedish holiday Valborg on April 30, but I had no interest in attending. We stayed at home. Then, a tragedy unfolded that day, something that should never take place but regrettably occurs with alarming frequency in this country. The news reported a fatal shooting at a pool party in San Diego, leaving several people with serious injuries.

It was terrible news, and it became even more devastating when I found out that one of the injured was one of my coworkers. I couldn't believe it. She was seriously injured and had been rushed to the hospital. The doctors were waiting for the swelling to go down so they could operate, but they said she would survive. But her friend didn't make it. Her three children would now have to grow up without their mom. The leniency of gun laws in this country made me furious. Even though tragedy after tragedy occurred, Republicans refused to discuss stricter regulations. This year was getting worse and worse.

10

THE ABORTION

The alarm clock beeped at seven, but I was already awake. The knot of tension in my gut had grown during the night, making it impossible to sleep. My thoughts raced. John took Juni to preschool, and I tried eating breakfast but had no appetite. I gave up on eating and sat down on the couch with my phone, searching for more answers to my questions about the abortion. There weren't many hours left now.

Our dog Leia jumped out of the car and happily ran into the doggie daycare when we dropped her off, blissfully unaware of where we were heading next. Neither John nor I knew where the abortion clinic was, so I navigated with directions from my phone. We didn't know where to park, but as we got closer, a security guard spotted us and pointed to the back of the building. The parking lot was empty. A few weeks later, my friend Liz told me she had driven past the clinic to see people protesting outside. She texted, *Ahh, I thought of you when I drove by Planned Parenthood ... and saw protesters. I got SO MAD!!* There were no protesters this morning, but that the security guard was necessary still made me uncomfortable. He nodded toward us and held the door open as we entered.

The security guard closed the door behind us, trapping us in a tiny room with bare walls and locked doors. I didn't know what I had expected, but it wasn't this. Looking straight ahead, we saw a small window. The receptionist pulled back a curtain so we could see and talk to her through the window, but she sat safely behind bulletproof glass. She asked for my ID, and I showed her my driver's license. She verified that my name was on the list of today's patients before unlocking the door to the waiting room.

I walked up to a second window, and just like at the first, the staff were sitting behind bulletproof glass. The woman behind the glass pointed to a phone receiver, and I picked it up so we could talk. The situation was surreal. Was this really happening to me? The security measures were palpable, and it was depressing to think about why they were needed.

The sun was shining outside but it didn't reach the waiting room. The blinds were down, presumably to make us feel safer, but it had the opposite effect. It only amplified the feeling that we needed to hide. A TV screen was showing the movie *The Holiday,* and now, I'm transported back to this moment every time that movie comes on. Posters asking for donations covered the walls, reminding me that if the Republicans got their way, no tax money would go to Planned Parenthood at all. Many patients rely on Planned Parenthood as their only affordable healthcare clinic.

It upset me that healthcare isn't a right in this country, but I was grateful that we lived in a liberal state. I was also thankful that there were no protesters outside and that the clinic was only a short fifteen-minute drive away. In many other states, patients weren't as fortunate.

John had never visited a Planned Parenthood clinic before. He told me he given a neighbor a ride to a clinic when he was in the Navy but hadn't gone inside. I had never been a patient here before, but I had gone with a friend to another of their clinics during college when she needed birth control. I didn't recall their security measures being so stringent back then—maybe they had to change due to increasing violence.

Even though we didn't have to wait that long, I had to go to the bathroom three times before they called my name. John wanted to come with me to the exam room, but they stopped him at the door. They asked me several times in the exam room to confirm that I wanted him to come. Of course I wanted him with me. It saddened me it's not a given for some people. Planned Parenthood's policy is always to ask questions to ensure you feel safe with your partner. The nurse went to get John, and when he came, he wore a sticker with his name on his shirt. The nurse measured my blood pressure and explained the process of the procedure. I received a painkiller, and they patiently answered our many questions, some more than once. Despite their efforts, they couldn't find a suitable vein in my left arm to draw blood. They wanted to save the best vein in my right arm for the following day. They managed to draw blood from my left hand, and I winced as they inserted the needle.

It was at that moment it truly sank in for John. He realized there was no going back and wanted it to be over so we could heal and move on. But it wasn't something we could get done quickly; this was just the first day.

I took off my pants and underwear, then lay on the narrow bed. I braced myself for the pain, but I wasn't ready for it to hurt as much as it did. Despite having given birth and suffered a second-degree burn, I had never felt pain like this before. As the doctor inserted nine seaweed sticks into the opening of the cervix, I screamed and squeezed John's hand. The sticks would absorb fluid from the body and slowly enlarge the opening to the cervix. Next, they placed a gauze pad inside the vagina to absorb blood and secure the sticks. Before inserting them, they showed me the seaweed sticks and gauze, but my tears made it impossible to see. They walked me through what they were doing, but I couldn't pay attention. The pain was excruciating, and I couldn't focus on anything else. The nurse asked if I needed a break, but I didn't want to extend the suffering. Through gritted teeth, I urged them to finish what they needed to do.

After the procedure, they told me I could get dressed and go home when I felt ready. I was dizzy and in pain, and my feet were so cold that I had lost feeling in them. The nurse applied an ice pack to my neck and placed a heating pad on my stomach to alleviate the nausea and pain.

It felt unthinkable that I could ever walk out of the clinic. I don't know how long I lay there, but eventually, with John's help, I managed to sit up. He helped me get dressed and took the bag with medicine and instructions, including a card with an emergency number and information about what they had done in case we had to call an ambulance at night. The nurse helped us to the front, and I waited with her and the security guard while John got the car from the parking lot. I needed their help to get into the front seat. The pain was indescribable. We stopped at a drive-through pharmacy on the way home to pick up painkillers, antibiotics, and iron tablets.

We came home, and John helped me up the stairs. Each step felt impossible. I made it to the second floor and sank into our most comfortable chair. The rest of the afternoon passed in a blurry haze. We had asked Sara and Eddie to pick up Leia at the doggie daycare and take care of her overnight. John ensured my painkillers were within reach before leaving to pick Juni up from preschool. She came home wondering what was wrong with me. It was difficult for a two-year-old to comprehend that a hug couldn't make the pain go away. Her tears came when she wasn't allowed to sit on my lap. We both cried.

The painkillers provided little relief. I wished I had been given something stronger. After dinner, I wasn't allowed to eat or drink anything else before the next stage of the abortion the following day. The night was a long battle with unbearable pain and a thirst I had never felt before. John helped me to and from the bathroom. Despite the lack of fluids, I had to go way too often.

Juni crawled into bed with us at six in the morning. The alarm clock blared fifteen minutes later. John took a quick shower before he helped Juni get ready for preschool and packed her lunch. I dressed in a black skirt, baggy shirt, and college sweater. We drove to the preschool right before seven. Juni knew we were going to the doctor because I wasn't feeling well. As we were leaving, we saw her standing in the doorway with a quivering chin and tears in her eyes. This wasn't our usual morning routine. I could feel my cheeks getting wet, too.

The security guard was once again standing outside the clinic when we arrived. We walked up to the bulletproof glass, and I showed the receptionist my driver's license. John filled out a form confirming that he was my driver. As a patient, you must have someone for transportation because you can't drive yourself afterward. The thought of women having no one to confide in was truly heartbreaking.

Several couples were already sitting in the waiting room; none of them looked married (at least, they did not have wedding rings on). There was also a young woman sitting there with her mother. The clinic mainly performed abortions on Wednesdays and judging by the expressions on everyone's faces, we were all there for the same reason. We were called in one by one. Today, John wasn't allowed to join me in the exam room; why, I didn't know, and I didn't think to question the rule.

I handed him my purse, gave him a quick hug and kiss, and walked in alone.

I ended up in the same exam room as the day before. A nurse fumbled putting on my patient information bracelet. She said this was the hardest thing she had done all day. It seemed like an absurd thing to say to a patient. I didn't know if she was being serious or ironic, and I didn't know how to answer. She tried to measure my blood pressure, but there was something wrong with the machine, so she went to get another one. The new machine worked. She asked me to take off my clothes and jewelry, everything but my underwear and bra. I was nervous about putting my wedding rings in the basket and wondered if this was why no one else in the waiting room was wearing them. I unbuttoned the gown too much and had to ask the nurse for help to get it on. She told me another nurse would arrive soon and left the room. I felt nauseous and dizzy and had to lie down. I wished John had been allowed to wait with me. I felt incredibly alone and didn't understand why he had to sit in the waiting room. I needed his strength and support more than ever.

The second nurse arrived to insert the IV. She still had issues finding a vein, even though they had saved the best arm for today. She gave me a blanket and left the room. I was shivering, and the world was spinning. I wrapped the blanket around myself. With tears streaming down my cheeks, I said "I'm sorry" and "goodbye" to a life that wouldn't be lived. There was no turning back.

After waiting for over an hour, I wondered if the next nurse had forgotten about me. When she finally arrived, she handed me a glass with a sour drink and told me to finish it; afterward, I couldn't remember why. She asked me to go to the bathroom when the glass was empty. Back in the exam room, it was only minutes until it was time to go to the operating room.

It finally became my turn, and once the nurse led me into

the next room, everything happened very quickly. I lay down on the operating table, and the nurse walked me through what would happen next. The anesthesiologist put a mask on me and adjusted the IV, and then the doctor entered the room.

"I'll be the one performing the abortion. Do you have any questions?" He didn't share his name. He glanced at my chart and said, "This is a very unusual diagnosis." All I could do was nod. It didn't take long for the anesthetic to kick in, and I drifted off.

When they nudged me back to consciousness, I was sitting in another room. I felt groggy, my brain in a fog, and I heard a nurse tell me I could sleep for thirty minutes. I didn't fall asleep, but I closed my eyes and rested. I heard other women being rolled into the same big room. Some had already woken up and were on their way out. Drapes for privacy separated us, and I overheard the woman next to me complain that she couldn't stop shaking, no matter how many blankets they put on her. I remembered this from the birth of my daughter, how I froze and shook uncontrollably, but I had forgotten what caused it.

After what I assumed was thirty minutes, a nurse came in and helped me to the bathroom. Each step was a challenge. I felt dizzy, my legs wobbly. The nurse brought the basket with my belongings. She checked how much I had bled into the pad I was wearing and asked if I could put my clothes on by myself. I said I could try, and she disappeared.

I sat down on the toilet and put on my underwear with a thick pad. I felt grateful for my outfit choice and was relieved to see my rings in the basket. In the hall, a nurse guided me to a chair and offered me water or Sprite, a granola bar, pretzels, or a lollipop. My throat was dry, and I gulped the water. I finished the glass and requested a refill. I declined the purple lollipop, guessing it was grape-flavored, so I asked for a different color. Then, they guided me to the entrance, where John was waiting.

He had been sitting in the waiting room the whole time, reading on his tablet, and watching TV. Still struggling to walk, I stayed with the nurse and security guard as John went to get the car.

We drove straight home. My appetite was gone. All I could get down were painkillers, some water, and a small chocolate bar my mom had sent from Sweden. I sat in the same comfy chair in our living room as the day before and watched an episode of *Midsomer Murders*. I couldn't stay awake any longer than that. After John helped me up to the bedroom, I took another dose of painkillers and dozed off.

I woke up when John came home with Juni and Leia. The girls ran upstairs and jumped on the bed. Leia licked my face while Juni questioned why I was in bed, urging me to come to the living room. When I went to the bathroom, I was shocked to find a bloody mess in my underwear. It wasn't your typical period. I changed the pad before I stumbled down the stairs and joined Juni on the couch. She was worried about me and didn't understand why I didn't feel better now that I had been to the doctor. I lay in bed at night with a heating pad on my stomach. It took a long time before I fell asleep.

11

AFTERWARD

The following day I took painkillers every four hours as instructed. Before lunch, I stepped into the shower on trembling legs for the first time since the abortion. The blood gushed out. I asked John to bring me toilet paper and pads. I needed to wipe off the blood before I got out of the tub.

I didn't move from the couch that evening, and Leia didn't leave my side. As the physical pain lessened, the emotional pain doubled. I had a difficult time finding relevant information and books about my type of abortion on the internet. Finding unbiased information free from religious or political influences was nearly impossible.

I faced another sleepless night. I emailed my supervisors in the morning and told them what had happened. Despite their religious beliefs, they were supportive and asked me to take the time off that I needed. One of them wrote: *My prayers are with you and your family. Let me know if I can do anything at all for you.* The other replied shortly after: *Linda, I'm so sorry to hear this news and keeping you in my thoughts and prayers. Please take the time you need as we understand how hard this must be. If you need anything please let us know. Thinking of you.*

Not having to worry about work was a relief. Some workplaces in this country wouldn't be as understanding. The company I used to work for was managed by older white Mormon men. I can only guess how they would have handled a situation like this.

Nature can be so cruel. When the weekend arrived, my milk had come in, causing my breasts to become large, lumpy, discolored, and painfully sensitive. I could only sleep on my back, which caused back pain as well. I lay on a heating pad and wore a nursing bra at night. I faithfully took the painkillers and hoped that I could get a few hours of sleep. To alleviate pain and reduce milk supply, I wrapped cabbage around my breasts and alternated with ice packs. The milk in my breasts was a sad reminder I didn't have a baby to nurse, nor would I have one. I discovered an online support group called Termination for Medical Reasons, where people shared similar experiences. It made me feel, however briefly, less alone.

The weekend ended, but the situation remained unchanged. The pain in my chest and back made it impossible to sleep, and my breasts looked abused. I remembered the difficulties I had when I breastfed Juni. Because of the pain and cramps, I extended my sick leave. I updated my out-of-office message and said I would return the following Monday. I would try to work before then, but I didn't want anyone to expect a response. The amount of work I had to do once I returned felt daunting.

The days passed, but my breasts showed no signs of change. There was no relief from the pain. I asked my doctor if he had any advice or could write a prescription. He was out of the office, but a nurse replied and recommended pseudoephedrine tablets, along with continuing with what I was already doing. John called various stores and found a shop that sold No More Milk tea, a remedy for reducing milk production. I heated water for the tea and swallowed the pseudoephedrine tablets with a sip of water when he got home.

It took another day for my breasts to realize there was no baby to feed. They were still lumpy and tender, but one breast was slightly smaller. I sipped my tea, took more medication, and still wrapped cabbage around my breasts, all in hopes of reducing my milk supply. The experience felt like déjà vu from when I stopped breastfeeding Juni.

I searched Swedish online bookstores and the Swedish library's ebooks for resources. Few discussed abortion. I found *The Toughest Round: A Personal Story About Abortion, Miscarriage, IVF And Egg Donation* by Åsa Sandell. I downloaded and read it. The book was worth reading, but it focused on IVF and egg donation, not abortion.

I couldn't find any books written by someone in my situation. Then the thought hit me—what if I wrote one? The idea scared me. I have been writing for as long as I can remember, but I had never completed a book manuscript. There were several unfinished drafts saved on my computer's hard drive. I feared this would be another unfinished book project. Opening up about what we had been through felt intimidating, for better or worse. I wasn't ashamed of what we had been through, but people could be cruel if they had differing opinions. I had read too many offensive comments and posts on the internet. The books I found in English were often judgmental. Even so, I wished I had been able to read about the experiences of someone in a similar situation. I would have to discuss it with John. He didn't know that I had been writing a diary. He probably thought I was writing the crime fiction novel I never finished. I made another cup of tea, sat down at the computer, and wrote while music played in the background. My tears flowed. Again.

On Thursday, I was back at work. I spoke to my Swedish colleague on the phone and ended the conversation with the Swedish expression, "We're not making any babies here," to convey the lack of progress. I realized it was true on multiple levels, and suddenly, the words felt sour. I promised myself never to use that expression again.

I received an invitation to a Mother's Day luncheon at Juni's preschool; they celebrated a few days in advance. I wasn't in the mood to be social, but I didn't want to disappoint Juni. I had done enough of that in the past few months. I showered and opened my closet, examining my wardrobe. I had been wearing nothing but yoga pants for the past few months, so I was unsure if anything else would fit. Before the abortion, I had a noticeable belly and had to wear maternity clothes. I tried on a pair of skinny jeans and successfully buttoned them. Even with my muffin top, it felt like a small victory. My breasts still hurt, but things were slowly going in the right direction, so I continued to drink tea and take the pseudoephedrine pills.

It was getting close to lunchtime, so I headed to the preschool. It was all worth it when I saw how happy it made Juni. She bounced up and down with excitement as she gave me the gift and hat she had made. What I wasn't prepared for, however, were the questions. "Do you have more children?" is a common question at social events like this one. I struggled to hold back the tears. I was sitting next to a mother who worked for a prominent conservative church nearby, and her constant references to God made me feel uneasy. I can only imagine her horror and judgment if I had told her about the abortion I had last week.

The children had prepared a few songs, and they recited a poem to all the mothers:

"Mommy, I love you, for all that you do. I'll kiss you and hug you, 'cause you love me too. You feed me and need me, to teach you to play. So smile 'cause I love you, on this Mother's Day."

When the hour was up, I hugged Juni tight, and I saw her lower lip quiver as I walked away. I exhaled as I escaped the other parents. I wasn't ready for social gatherings yet. I would hug and kiss Juni a little extra when she came home this afternoon.

Back at my work computer, I admired the bracelet she had made for me, and I felt fortunate that I got to be her mom. This time, I shed happy tears.

In the afternoon, I started bleeding heavily. I took a short walk with the family, and when we got home, I felt a sudden rush of blood, and the cramps came back. Once again, I turned to the internet, and it wasn't all that uncommon based on the articles I read. Many had similar concerns and raised the same questions. I took it easy the rest of the day. After Juni fell asleep, we watched TV. At least the pregnancy fatigue was gone.

In the United States, Mother's Day is celebrated two weeks before the holiday in Sweden. The card Juni and John gave me the morning of the American Mother's Day brought tears to my eyes. I loved my little family. We had brunch at a New Zealand restaurant nearby. It had been a long time since I had been out to eat with my family. Later, a bouquet arrived from my brother-in-law and sister-in-law, and I received several text messages and calls.

I empathized with all the mothers and women who, for different reasons, are reminded of children they had, couldn't have, or chose not to have. It must be one of the toughest days of the year for them. In the United States, one in four pregnancies ends in miscarriage, about 12 percent of couples struggle with infertility problems, and each year, around 24,000 infants die before their first birthday. All these people are grieving. On a day like Mother's Day, it's difficult to find the right words to say to them. Therefore, people rarely say anything. But the silence also hurts. The longing for a child doesn't go away. I didn't know how I would cope with it.

My sister had a miscarriage after she gave birth to her first child, and when I told her about our situation, she said that the grief will fade with time, but it will never disappear.

I slept poorly, as usual. Juni came to us sometime during the night to cuddle in our bed. I didn't know what time it was, but the morning was still far away. She had had a nightmare and didn't want to stay in her bed. We didn't have the heart to force her away, so for the rest of the night, she lay close to me.

I lay awake worrying about if and how I would change as a parent from what we had been through. I was already worrying more than usual that something would happen to Juni. I didn't want to become overly protective or try to stop her from exploring the world. Then I wondered if I would swing in the other direction and let her get away with more things. She had come to me in our bed in the middle of the night, which she had never done before. I hugged her as she stretched out, taking up more space than a tiny human should. When she talked in her sleep and mumbled, "I'm making coffee," my heart overflowed with love.

The weekend came, and we took a trip to Ikea. I tried to pretend everything was normal, but it was difficult when the cramps constantly reminded me of everything that had happened. After shopping, we picked up lunch at a Mexican restaurant and brought it to Sara and Eddie's house. They had a little over two weeks left until their estimated due date. My heart stung when I saw all the baby clothes in their nursery.

On Norway's Independence Day, May 17, it was two weeks since we terminated the pregnancy. It was two weeks since we had the abortion. Few in the United States used that word. I saw that some online forums suggested saying "voluntary termination of pregnancy" because the word "abortion" is so taboo. Others disagreed and argued that using the word abortion would help destigmatize women's rights to make decisions about their bodies. If we who have had an abortion are afraid to say the word or talk about it, what message does that send to those around us?

It's difficult to change society. A woman's right to choose includes the right to not share her experiences if she doesn't want to. But if we collectively refuse to talk about abortion openly, if we hide it and use other words instead, how can change ever happen?

I was guilty myself. When I talked about our decision and what we had done, I usually said that we had terminated the pregnancy rather than say that we had an abortion. When I looked through what I had written in my journal entries, I often referred to it as "the procedure" instead of "abortion." I decided I would go back and edit that. However, for me, it was more important that we talked about abortion than what words were used when we talked about it. For some, the word abortion implies that one wanted to end the pregnancy, which was misleading when it was done for medical reasons. But the more I read, the more often I used the word abortion because abortion means ending a pregnancy for whatever reason. I wondered if it was different in Sweden. I couldn't remember people avoiding the word, but I had had no real reason to discuss it before.

If we hadn't had an abortion, I would have been in week 21, more than halfway through the pregnancy. Instead, life had taken a different turn, and I was back to wearing my regular pants.

I had Monday off, so I started cleaning and organizing the

garage to keep my mind busy. I had forgotten about all the baby items we kept in there. I tried my best not to look at the crib, the changing table, the bathtub. The garbage container gradually filled up as I cleaned. The baby things remained untouched.

I wrote in the afternoon. It helped to put my feelings into words. With each word I wrote, I fought against the taboo of my situation. I wanted to write in capital letters that my grief was as valid as other types of grief. I wanted to scream out loud to make people understand the pain I was going through. But I wrote instead. I wrote to get all my feelings down on paper and, hopefully, to show others they aren't alone. I didn't mind sharing my story with strangers, but I worried about my family and friends reading about the most private thing I have ever been through. What would they think?

But at the same time, that was the core of the problem. I didn't want to feel that nervousness. I shouldn't have to worry, and neither should anyone else.

I told John about getting all my feelings down on paper to process my grief. He gave me his full support, and even though I had expected it, it was still a relief to hear. But since the subject was so taboo, I wasn't sure he wanted me to share it with the world. It wasn't exactly something you mentioned in your Facebook status. Or did you? Should I?

John admitted he had mixed feelings about me sharing my story. He knew I processed my emotions through writing and understood it would be therapeutic. At the same time, he worried about potential harassment from abortion opponents. John hoped the response would be less vitriolic since I was writing in Swedish. Sweden's approach to reproductive rights differed significantly from the United States. He was also nervous that his relatives would discover my writing and judge us, but he quickly overcame that. During a crisis, it becomes apparent what matters in your life. He made it clear that his focus was on us and our family, and he assured me it was more important for him to support me than to uphold a façade to relatives he rarely saw.

We had a follow-up appointment with Dr. Robertson scheduled for the following day. We hoped that my body had healed as it should—I was still bleeding some, but it was no longer the bloodbath it had been. I knew my broken heart would take significantly longer to heal, if ever. John patiently listened to all my thoughts and feelings. We had decided that we wouldn't consider trying for a second child until after the summer. After such a life-changing experience, we recognized it would be wise to pause big life decisions. But I didn't want to wait any longer than that. Either the roller coaster would start over again, or we would donate all the baby items.

I was happy and grateful that we had each other in our little family. As a Swede living abroad, I sometimes felt I didn't have a sense of belonging anywhere. When I expressed that feeling, John reassured me that I truly belonged to our family, and I knew he was right. I thought of an acquaintance whose husband betrayed her and their son with lies and infidelity. It could always be worse.

I talked to Sara, who had just been to her last prenatal appointment before giving birth. She told me how painful the exam was. It reminded me of my experience with that type of pain. As the holiday weekend neared, she knew that if her baby didn't arrive soon, she would be induced. Soon, their child would be here. Juni eagerly awaited the baby's arrival. I felt anxious because many things had gone awry this year. Their birth had to go right. Perhaps the Swedish World Cup gold in ice hockey was the event that reversed the trend of bad news. At least, I hoped so.

The weekend came and the weather in Southern California was warm and sunny, not the usual cloudy "May Gray." Liz and

Pat's daughter Emilia turned two, and they had invited us to a *Finding Dory*-themed birthday party in the park. We headed to the beach once the party was over. I couldn't remember the last time I had spent that much time outdoors. Juni asked if I felt better, and I answered, "A little," but without any conviction.

At the end of May, I logged on to the computer to see an email from my medical group's health portal. They had updated my medical records. I logged into my account and saw that they had deactivated the pregnancy and chromosomal abnormality diagnoses and added that I had had a surgical procedure—an abortion. Black on white. There it was. One by one, the symptoms disappeared, and soon, a hole in my heart would be the only thing left. Was there a diagnosis code for that?

I tried to hold back tears as I entered the clinic for the follow-up appointment with Dr. Robertson. The nurse didn't know what to say when she saw me. She attempted to make a joke about John stepping up on the scale after I weighed myself. She measured my blood pressure and left the room. When Dr. Robertson came in, he walked over and hugged me. He asked how I was doing, and his kindness released the floodgates. It took some time before I could answer. He handed me some tissues, and we discussed the abortion, healing, and the future. He examined me and gave me the green light to return to my regular routine. Then he said that the bleeding would stop soon and to expect my period to resume in mid-June. We talked about birth control and the probabilities of genetic abnormalities and miscarriages. He said I could call whenever I wanted and hugged me again before he moved on to the next patient.

In the car on the way home, John and I talked about how misleading all the data we had reviewed was. The probabilities were based on amniocentesis results; not everyone did that test, and not all miscarriages were included either. I understood there was no choice but to settle for the available information. Still, knowing that the statistics didn't show the complete picture was essential. Regardless of what the actual risk was, my age was against me. First, getting pregnant, then not having a miscarriage, and then having a healthy child who survived. Could I even consider it?

Dr. Robertson told me to enjoy the spring and summer before we made any decisions. I agreed I would try. I was standing in the checkout line at the grocery store later in the day when it hit me that the pregnancy was over. No more doctor visits were on the calendar, and my medical records no longer listed the diagnosis. Most people didn't even know it ever existed.

12

DISENFRANCHISED GRIEF

I was still searching for information on the internet on everything related to abortions, even though it felt like I had read most of it already. There was information for people who had had miscarriages, and I saw a book called *Miscarriage: The Right to Grieve.* There were books, keepsakes, and non-judgmental information. They had every right to grieve. Miscarriage was a terrible thing to go through.

But I had a right to grieve, too. I found little information about my situation, and what I did find was often judgmental. Some argued that since abortion was something you chose, you opted out of the right to grieve. Processing my grief felt even more complicated when many in society saw it as shameful and didn't take it seriously.

I saw on Facebook that an acquaintance's father had died. It was heartbreaking, but I envied that the tragedy was so natural and accepted to share on social media and to receive all the love and kind messages from family and friends. You wanted that support. You needed that support. But those who struggle with disenfranchised grief so rarely get it.

Disenfranchised grief isn't discussed, socially accepted, or observed by society. Examples of disenfranchised grief include miscarriage, abortion, suicide, or the death of a former partner. The loss is real, but people often feel that they don't have the same right to grieve as people experiencing other forms of grief. You suffer, but you can't share your pain. The secrecy makes it extra challenging to move on. Women who choose to have an abortion often become isolated, leaving them even less inclined to talk about it. This silence is true in American society.

Even though I had only been treated kindly so far, I was still hesitant to share my abortion experience. I worried about how people would react. I shared no details even though I wanted to; some still became noticeably uncomfortable. It felt like many wanted to change the subject as quickly as possible.

"Grief work" is an appropriate term because it's hard. Lack of support makes things even harder, a sad reality for many. After an abortion, there is no ritual to process the grief. But for women whose abortions were painful and emotional decisions, grief follows the same stages: denial, anger, negotiation, depression, and acceptance. I couldn't imagine ever getting to the final stage.

How could I move on? When would life become normal? Would it ever be normal again? I wanted a keepsake because I wouldn't get a push present this time. After the birth of my daughter, I received a beautiful necklace. This time, I had my eyes on a ring with a sapphire gemstone. The due date was September, and sapphire is September's birthstone. I would have to wait to justify the expense, maybe when John found a full-time job again.

Mizuko kuyō is a traditional Buddhist ceremony in Japan for children who weren't born because of miscarriage, stillbirth, or abortion. *Mizuko* translates to "water baby," a term used in Japanese to describe a deceased fetus or child, while *kuyō* denotes a memorial ceremony. The ceremony may take different forms, but it typically involves prayers and offerings of candles, flowers, and incense. The ritual makes the abortion visible and aids in moving on. I wished I had such an outlet for my grief. Abortion is considered a sin in many religions, compelling women to conceal it and grieve in silence.

I came across a company on Instagram that offered ultrasound watercolor paintings. I clicked through to their website since the ultrasound photos were all we had. It felt like a respectful way to honor a life that didn't exist. I pulled out the pictures of my ultrasounds and realized I had never looked at the ones that were taken the same day we did the amniocentesis. I slowly flipped through them, and my heart broke into a thousand more pieces, seeing the fetus that never became a baby. Even though I didn't regret the decision, it still hurt. The loss of what I thought our family would become was devastating. I cried my way through the evening, and the ultrasound images will be etched in my memory forever. John didn't look at them until much later.

We spent our Sunday morning with friends at Sara and Eddie's, hanging out by the pool. Later, our whole family took a nap at home. That evening, we welcomed our friends Will, Ashley, and their son Mason for dinner. They already knew about the abortion. Will shared his childhood experience of going to protests outside abortion clinics with his conservative parents. When they shouted, "Abortion clinics must go!" he thought they were saying, "Martian clinics must go." The experience was both exciting and confusing for a little boy. Will couldn't understand why anyone wanted clinics for aliens from Mars. As an adult, he held views differing from those of his parents, but he chose not to discuss politics with them to avoid conflict.

Ashley shared how her brother and his wife recently experienced a stillbirth at week 39. Despite the NIPT test showing no risks, the woman stopped feeling any kicks a week before the estimated due date. They had received a false negative result, and the fetus had chromosomal abnormalities. False negative results are rare, but they can happen. The couple already had a daughter. Soon, they would have a memorial service for the fetus that died in the womb. There were so many of us who were grieving for different reasons, but with the same result. So many people had sad experiences; when I shared mine, others seemed more willing and comfortable sharing theirs.

I continued to organize and clean out the house and garage. I focused on the task at hand to stop all the thoughts that were otherwise plaguing me. We moved in when Juni was seven months old and hadn't cleared anything out since then. The garage still contained plenty of baby items and furniture. We had only gotten rid of the things we didn't want or wouldn't use if we ever had a second child.

I had read Marie Kondo's books about how to only keep things that bring you joy. It was more complex to implement in real life, but I did my best. Material things didn't matter. All I needed in life was Juni, John, and Leia.

We received news that Sara and Eddie had checked in at the hospital, and their daughter was born in the evening the following day. It had been a long journey for them. They couldn't conceive naturally, and their IVF attempts in the United States failed. Ultimately, an IVF clinic in Sweden made their dream of becoming parents a reality. I was thrilled for them, but I couldn't help but think about our situation. We were only four months away from what would've been our estimated due date.

We visited them the day after they came home from the hospital. I had forgotten how tiny newborns can be. Juni, who was about to turn three, looked gigantic in comparison. As I looked at the little girl, I felt the tears welling up. I fought to keep them away. This moment was about them, about their happiness, not about me. I thought of a poem my grandmother had put up on her kitchen wall after my grandfather's passing: "My eyes may sparkle, my lips may smile, but no one can see the tears in my heart." My heart ached when I saw Juni with the baby. She was so careful and gentle. She would have loved to help with a little sister.

We visited Sara and Eddie again when their daughter was a week old. Seeing their happiness made me genuinely happy, but the loss of our unborn daughter was immense, and the hole in my heart grew.

I desperately wanted to be a good friend to Sara during this exciting time. She has always been the friend who calls, asks all the right questions, and is understanding and supportive. I hoped I gave that to her, too. But at home, I cried. By this point, I would have been much more than halfway through the pregnancy, looking forward to the fall and the time after my daughter would have been born. Now, I dreaded it. Despite knowing we made the right choice, my heart sometimes disagreed.

However, I knew it would have been worse if we hadn't made our decision. I would have been filled with anxiety and fear about adjusting to a new life. What I grieved was the reality I thought we would get when the pregnancy test was positive and before the NIPT results came. But sadly, that was never an option for us. Thankfully, we already had the most wonderful daughter imaginable. Juni is bright, kind, beautiful, and stubborn, with solid leadership qualities. But I grieved that I couldn't give her a sister. Maybe we could give her other things instead. We could try to travel more and show her the world. She said our dog was her sister, and they would tease each other as only siblings could.

On a family walk, Juni kept chatting as usual, and this day, she talked about her imaginary sister's name. She didn't know how close she was to reality, and her speculations about a make-believe sister made my heart ache. John glanced at me with a worried look in his eye. I pretended I didn't hear what she said and changed the subject, but Juni wouldn't stop talking about it.

My friend Anne, who had the same health insurance as me, offered to call the company and ask about mental health resource coverage. I thanked her but declined. I didn't know why. It probably would have been good for me. Instead, I kept writing. It had become my therapy. I imagined I was writing the book to help others in the same situation, but the truth was that I was writing for my own sake. I wrote to cope with my grief, find a sense of purpose, and make sense of our experience. I wasn't sure if anyone would ever get to read what I wrote.

One evening, John and I watched Chelsea Handler's talk show. Her guests were comedian Sarah Silverman and the president of Planned Parenthood, Cecile Richards. It was a relief that someone finally brought up the elephant in the room. John looked up an article Cecile Richards had written, and I felt such a sense of recognition. She said that if a woman is relieved after an abortion, she is labeled as heartless and without emotion—but if she feels remorse and loss, her emotions are used to manipulate the abortion law debate. Therefore, we remain silent. Women don't talk about their abortions because of the fear of being labeled irresponsible and selfish, and facing intrusive and judgmental inquiries. As a woman, you should never have to defend or explain your decision.

It was only when Cecile Richards became the president of Planned Parenthood that she revealed her personal abortion story. Together, she and the organization worked to end the silence that fueled the stigma around abortion. We wanted to achieve the same thing. Unfortunately, the United States had a president who made decisions that hurt women's healthcare in unprecedented ways. Many of President Trump's actions focused on undoing the progress accomplished by President Obama.

Because Planned Parenthood provides women access to abortions, they have long been the target of Republican attacks, and these attacks intensified during President Trump's administration. Trump and the Republicans repealed the rule that Obama put in place, which stated that it's against the law for states to block people from accessing healthcare at organizations that also provide abortions. Under the Trump administration, states could once again withhold funding from Planned Parenthood.

Trump also proposed replacing the Affordable Care Act, passed during the Obama administration, with the American Health Care Act, which would jeopardize women's healthcare coverage. To satisfy the religious groups that supported Trump's election, coverage for prenatal care and contraception would be eliminated. Trump's views on abortion rights had conveniently evolved as he acknowledged the significant impact of the conservative religious right on voter turnout and election outcomes.

Republicans also reinstated the Global Gag Rule, which withheld federal funds from international health organizations that offered abortion services, even in countries where it was legal. President Reagan initially introduced the rule, and every Republican president has renewed or reintroduced it since then.

Transgender individuals who had bravely served their country were once again barred from military service despite President Obama's previous decision to allow them to serve. President Trump didn't value their service.

President Trump not only excused and defended men accused of sexual harassment, but he himself faced multiple accusations, which he denied, adding to the burden women already face with sexual harassment. On top of that, he helped repeal laws that helped universities handle sexual abuse cases.

President Trump's initial budget proposal faced controversy because of funding cuts for federal programs like Women, Infants and Children (WIC), which provided food for impoverished women and children. Many Republicans claim to be pro-life but refuse to support children once they are born. It's impossible to believe their argument, given their contradictory actions.

Donald Trump and some Republicans also tried to stop the abortion that Jane Doe, a seventeen-year-old undocumented immigrant, sought to get in late 2017. She discovered her pregnancy a month after crossing the border into the United States. Jane Doe never wavered in her decision. Despite this, Republicans tried to block it with the help of the courts, which delayed the abortion. Their actions forced her to be pregnant several weeks longer than necessary. Many similar cases would follow it.

In Sweden, healthcare is accessible to all EU citizens, and everyone has the right to "care that cannot be deferred," including abortion and prenatal care.

Life and work carried on. One day, I attended a work meeting with a supervisor who knew about my situation. Afterward, I thanked her for her support. She had dealt with a lot of grief herself because of her daughter's suicide a few years earlier, and when I expressed my gratitude, she gave me a big hug. My tears flowed, and so did hers. "You should always bring tissues," she advised. I nodded. She also noted that as time went on, your days would become better. I hoped that would be true.

A few days later, I went to a work meeting with another person who knew about my abortion. I avoided talking to her as long as possible; I was nervous about how I would react. But when the meeting was over, and people were chatting in different groups, I thanked her for her support. She said she prayed for me and told me she had given birth to a child who died shortly after delivery. The baby had no limbs, but that wasn't known before the birth. It had all come as a shock to her. We cried together. I noticed some other coworkers looking at us, but I ignored them. I realized that when I shared my story, others felt comfortable to share theirs. Another colleague had a daughter who lived into adulthood; she was disabled and required constant care. These women were unaware of their children's issues before birth. None of them knew what they would've done if they had known.

One of my favorite movies when I was younger was *Dirty Dancing*. What I didn't think about at the time was that the film's central theme was abortion. It drives the story forward and exposes the harsh reality faced by women who have no choice but to resort to illegal abortions. I found it impossible to comprehend that many Republicans wanted to return to this reality. But just like the movie character Robbie, they only thought about themselves. To Robbie, it was unthinkable that he would have to deal with the consequences of sex.

We hear time and time again how Republican men who strongly oppose abortion conveniently shift their views when their mistress gets pregnant. An example of this was Tim Murphy, a congressman from Pennsylvania. He aligned fiercely with anti-abortion rhetoric but asked his mistress to have an abortion when he thought she was pregnant. Scott DesJarlais was another Republican politician who supported his ex-wife when she terminated two pregnancies and pressured a twenty-four-year-old woman with whom he had an affair to do the same. Despite their own experiences, they continued to oppose abortion for others. Empathy was missing, and all that remained was hypocrisy.

After a morning at the Birch Aquarium, the whole family fell asleep during Juni's naptime. In the afternoon, we drew with chalk on the sidewalk outside our front door. It was in the same location where a neighbor had fatally shot a man almost a year ago. The former neighbor was now serving a lengthy prison sentence. As we drew flowers and rainbows near the site of a man's death, I couldn't help but be reminded of the stark contrasts and overwhelming sadness and pain. I picked Leia up from doggie daycare and listened to the country channel. True to form, the lyrics expressed profound emotion. I didn't even try to stop the tears.

My close friend Henrik came over for dinner. He had recovered from his surgery, and we were happy to see him again. He was like a brother. We could talk about anything and everything. I was grateful for the support he had lent me throughout all that we had been through, from sending flowers the day after the abortion to always being there when I needed to talk.

I thought of Juni and hoped she might find a sister or brother someday. Sometimes, friends truly become family. I also hope that Juni can talk about anything without feeling ashamed, no matter what happens. I never want her to feel silenced.

John attended the Father's Day lunch organized by Juni's preschool. My heart overflowed with love, knowing I had these two. Father's Day wasn't as painful as Mother's Day, but I still cried. I cried over the fact that John, who was an exceptional father, wouldn't have two daughters this fall. He would've loved to have more than one child and handled it so well. He didn't struggle with this preschool event as much as I had, but it wasn't in his body that life had grown, either. His sadness and grief were valid, but he could distance himself differently than I could.

I started bleeding, and I hoped it was my period returning. It came earlier than my doctor had predicted, but who knew how my body worked? Everyone was different. It was another step closer to everything being "normal."

In the days that followed, I had severe stomach cramps. I hoped it was because of my period, but I didn't know. The pain disrupted my sleep, and I felt a bit off when I got up in the morning. I spent a few hours in front of the computer but didn't accomplish anything. I needed to rest, so I returned to bed and set the alarm for an hour. When it rang, I had a fever, headache, upset stomach, and joint pain. I had to take the rest of the day off; there was no other option. I slept all afternoon until Juni came home from preschool. I still felt sick and stayed on the couch for the rest of the evening. Hadn't I had enough trouble and pain this year?

My only symptom the following day was a stomachache, but I took another sick day. I worried the pain was related to the abortion. I couldn't tell whether the pain was in my stomach, uterus, or elsewhere. I wanted to give it more time before jumping to conclusions.

No one who had known what I had been through asked how I was doing anymore. Two months had passed since the abortion. Was that how long the statute of limitations was for my pain to be valid? It seemed to be the norm to pretend nothing had happened. Ignore the pregnancy, ignore the abortion, ignore the sadness and the emptiness. Act strong and put on a happy face. But that would have been a lie.

We could have pretended that I had only been pregnant once, that I had never had an abortion. I had become good at acting, so it was an option. Considering how many women have had abortions and how rarely people talk about it, it seems common to hide the truth. Someone even suggested we could say we had a miscarriage. It upset me, even though I knew they meant well. I assumed they thought we wanted to avoid questions about the abortion. I came across an article about a Canadian couple who had an abortion, and the husband's workplace had sent flowers to "the wife who had a miscarriage." Many people probably choose not to tell the truth, but I didn't want to be one of them.

I read the book *Tribe* by Sebastian Junger. He discusses how individuals with post-traumatic stress disorder find recovery easier when surrounded by a supportive community. People who have had an abortion often keep their experience to themselves, and, as a result, some of them may lack the support they need. Judgment instead of support makes the recovery process longer than it should be. Understanding and supporting family, friends, and coworkers could make the situation easier.

13

WE NEED TO TALK ABOUT ABORTION

Abortion is a politically controversial subject, especially in the United States. There are many people on both sides of the debate who make their voices heard, but the perspectives of women who have had abortions are often overlooked. We need to fix that; we need to talk about abortion. We must speak if we want things to change. We can't worry about what people think.

In the end, the abortion was my decision, and there was nothing wrong with that. It also wasn't bad that I was sad—feeling sad didn't mean that I regretted the abortion. Choosing to tell people about my abortion in this book was a somewhat controversial decision. Part of me thought seeing how people would react would be interesting. Maybe they wouldn't react at all. After all, Sweden and the United States were vastly different countries (the first edition of this book was only published in Swedish). But people need to share and talk about abortions everywhere.

I wanted to share my experience with more people. I wish I had been open about my pregnancy and everything that happened from the start. Then, I wouldn't feel like I had to pretend. But could I share it now, beyond the small circle of trust I had already told? The way I felt about sharing my story had changed, and I suspected it was part of the grieving and healing process. I wanted to tell people to ease my pain and sorrow, and I hoped my story might help others in the same situation feel less alone. If abortion hadn't carried such a stigma, my perspective might have been different from the beginning. Perhaps it would have been natural to talk about it then. It would've saved me a lot of tears.

Talking about topics related to the female body and pregnancies is often considered taboo. From miscarriage to regretting parenthood, the list includes a wide range of topics such as abortion, prenatal testing, infertility, and postpartum depression. The list also includes the grief that can sometimes accompany an abortion.

When it came to talking about abortion, there was nothing and no one that could silence me. Yet, I needed to brace myself for any possible response, and I wasn't sure if I was ready. But by avoiding discussions about abortion, we perpetuate its stigma and keep the harmful cycle going.

After work, Sara had invited Anne, Liz, and me for a happy hour. I arrived first. I worried about my emotions, but seeing Sara's baby this time went better, and I didn't feel as broken. I held the baby in my arms and rocked her back and forth.

When Liz and Anne arrived, we sat down at the table that Sara had already set. She opened the fridge and took out a bottle of Pinot Grigio, and she was about to pour it into our wine glasses when Anne raised her hand.

"Nothing for me, please," she said.

We looked at her, and it felt like the rug was pulled from under me when I realized she was pregnant. She already had two children, and they conceived their second child with IVF. I tried to collect myself and took a deep breath before saying,

"That's great news. Congratulations! I'll have a glass of wine for you, too." I gulped my wine to numb the pain. At the same time, I felt for her. I knew she was nervous about how it would go. Anne was a year older than me, and the odds weren't as favorable as they had been ten years ago. She was in week 10, and they had only told us so far.

Anne was the one who had offered to call our health insurance company to find out about mental health coverage. Did she worry about my reaction to this news? I didn't know. It didn't matter.

Sara said it was great that she could give outgrown clothes and toys to Anne now. I wanted to shout *"No*, give them to me!" But we wouldn't need any baby clothes. I thought about the boxes in the closet that I had saved. I didn't know what to do with them.

Anne gave me a ride home, and when we got to my house, she got out of the car and hugged me. Juni was already asleep, so when I got inside, I sat on the couch with a tissue in my hand and told John. He hugged me tight. The following day, I woke up with swollen eyes.

The next day, a letter from the specialist's office was waiting in our mailbox. My heart skipped a beat. What did they want? I opened the envelope and unfolded the paper—a bill. Ultrasound, $425. Amniocentesis, $750. Surgical tray, $10. My health insurance covered all but $20. Why didn't they charge me during our office visit instead of sending a sad reminder much later? I received a bill for $60 from my doctor even later and another bill from Planned Parenthood for $300. The total payment was $380, but the most significant payment was in tears.

I spoke to Jenny, who had had the miscarriage, and she had forgotten to cancel all her future doctor's appointments after her miscarriage. She ended up receiving a letter reminding her of the 18-week ultrasound—a heartbreaking reminder.

Three years prior, my contractions had started with Juni in my belly. But then I wasn't sure if they were contractions, and they were so infrequent that John still went to work. This year, I was sitting on the couch, drinking my morning coffee with my almost three-year-old girl sitting next to me, sniffling with a cold. She complained her nose hurt and her eyes were sad. She hadn't been sick in months, and now it hit her just in time for her *farmor* (grandmother), *farfar* (grandfather), *farbror* (uncle) Thomas, and *faster* (aunt) Megan to visit for her birthday. We had a birthday party with twenty people planned for the next day, and we didn't want to cancel. Juni had been excited about the party for weeks. She wanted a strawberry cake and yellow balloons. I texted everyone we had invited to let them know that the party would go ahead as planned but that the birthday girl had caught a cold. All the guests were going to come anyway.

My in-laws were on their way, and I was nervous. I hadn't spoken to them since the abortion, and I was still disappointed that my mother-in-law had told her sister about the pregnancy before we had given the go-ahead. They would be here in a few hours. I wondered how the weekend would be. According to John, they supported our decision but still saw abortion as a taboo subject and something not to be talked about.

We were going to have a pool party with Juni's favorite food —quesadillas—on the menu. We had picked up the strawberry cake, and the yellow balloons were in place. The clouds hung heavy until a couple of minutes before the party started, then the clouds parted, and the clear blue sky took over. My heart overflowed with happiness and gratitude when I saw Juni's happiness, almost forgetting she had a cold.

Juni fell asleep after the party, and we had to remind her of the presents she hadn't opened for her to wake up. The memories of three years ago when she was born, and the mixture of pain and joy I felt, came rushing back. I loved her more than anything in the world. But my heart also ached when I thought about the fact that there would be no contractions this fall.

The following day, we had dinner with John's brother, Thomas, and his wife, Megan. We went to Costa Brava, the Spanish tapas restaurant where we had our wedding dinner six years earlier. I took a deep breath and told them about the abortion. They were surprised that I was referred to Planned Parenthood. They had assumed that my medical group would perform the abortion. Unfortunately, in many places in this country, doctor's offices could be targeted with harassment if they provided them. They supported our decision, and I felt relieved after sharing my feelings.

I read an article about a woman who reached out to her gynecologist under the assumption that they could offer abortion services. After all, it's a standard and safe procedure. She was surprised when the answer was no. However, because of its political controversy, many doctors, hospitals, and medical groups refuse to perform abortions to shield themselves from protests.

The weekend went by, and my in-laws didn't mention the pregnancy or the abortion. I suspected they thought that was what I wanted. I wanted to shout that I wanted and needed to talk about the abortion. It only came up when John's mother asked if we would attend John's cousin's wedding in September. I said John could go, but I didn't know if I could. The wedding would be a week before what had been our due date. My voice cracked, and she said she understood and changed the subject.

We returned the baby mobile that John had as a child, which my in-laws had given to us when Juni was born. We said we wouldn't need it again. My mother-in-law took the bag without saying a word. Before they left, we also gave back the tricycle from the eighties that Juni had outgrown.

My phone pinged. Sara had sent a text message saying that one of her sister's friends in Sweden was pregnant but that they had found out there was a high risk of chromosomal abnormalities. They had received the result from the combined ultrasound and blood test, and now they were awaiting the NIPT test result. I told Sara that she could tell them about our experience and that her friend was welcome to contact me if she wanted to talk. I wished I had someone to talk to, and if I could help someone, I would be more than happy to do so. The couple had said they intended to have an abortion if the results showed chromosomal abnormalities. I reminded Sara that NIPT doesn't give a diagnosis, and she said she thought the couple would do amniocentesis if the NIPT showed risks as well. I hoped this was one time the test had given a false positive.

When the Swedish couple got their NIPT result, it showed no risk of chromosomal abnormalities, which was an immense relief. I was glad for them but couldn't stop thinking about our situation. Why were we so unlucky? Anne was still waiting for the result of her NIPT test. She was a year older than me, so age played a role in the risk, but despite that, there's usually a better chance of having a healthy child than not.

When Anne finally got the NIPT result, it was good news, and they also found out they were expecting a boy. I was happy for them, but I still battled with jealousy. I couldn't control it. I would've had a big belly by now if things had gone differently. Anne asked me if we would try again for a child, but I didn't want to talk anymore. We ended the call.

I knew people who had disabilities. They were active in various organizations and often posted on social media, which was completely understandable. I would have done the same if we had continued the pregnancy and given birth to a child with a chromosomal abnormality. Now, I focused my efforts on another critical issue: abortion rights. John was also more involved—he listened to all the podcasts about abortion he could find to hear what they had to say.

Regardless of your place in society, there will always be important matters to stand up for. But no one has the time or energy to deal with every issue. As a result, individuals tend to prioritize the problems that have a personal impact. This becomes especially clear in a society like the United States, where people must fend for themselves differently. Sweden is globally recognized for its high ranking in equality and its social safety net, with no current threats to abortion rights. But that could change. We must never take any rights for granted.

John and I had started watching *Sex and the City* after Juni's bedtime. Typically, we would watch one or two episodes each night. We had made it to season four and watched the episode "Coulda, Woulda, Shoulda." The story revolves around Charlotte's difficulties conceiving, Miranda's unexpected pregnancy, her considerations of abortion, and Carrie's abortion at twenty-two. The episode deeply resonated with me—the emotions, the envy, the difficult choices, and their repercussions.

In another episode, "Catch-38", Carrie was thirty-eight years old and in a relationship where she wouldn't have children. I faced a different dilemma at thirty-eight, not knowing if we would try for a second child. I felt old, even though I wasn't.

Although there was some recognition in the episodes, there is a problem with how television and film depict abortions. The University of California San Francisco conducted a research program on how media portrays abortion. The study found that abortion complications are much more common on television and film than in real life. They exaggerate not only the frequency but also the severity of such complications. Abortion is frequently depicted as dangerous and extreme, potentially causing infertility and depression. But in real life, such damning outcomes are extremely rare. Sometimes, there's grief involved, sometimes just a sense of relief. Abortion is a legal, safe procedure that improves women's health and lives. While screenwriters have the power to create drama on the big screen, the media plays a significant role in shaping our perception. Realistic portrayals of abortion are necessary for dispelling misconceptions about the procedure.

I got my period again, experienced heavy bleeding, and stayed home all day. I was grateful to have that option. My thinking wasn't rational, and I was on the verge of tears the entire time. I hoped my cycle would eventually return to how it was before the abortion.

After a couple of tough days with massive bleeding, chaotic hormones, and a rollercoaster of emotions, Jenny sent me a text message. She was pregnant again. She felt nauseous and described it as disgusting. Although she was worried about the outcome, there was a heartbeat this time, which provided some relief.

Following the news of Jenny's pregnancy, John and I discussed our future. We had two months left until what would've been the due date, but instead, we had to decide whether to start over. John said that right after the abortion, he wanted to try again but that he didn't want to say anything to pressure me then. Now, a while later, he wasn't so sure. We had the same doubts as before and even more reasons for concern. We were older and had already gone through nearly half a pregnancy with a fetus that had a chromosomal abnormality. Could we do it again, and would our relationship survive a second abortion? I felt a deep sadness and disappointment over all that had happened.

We decided to postpone the decision. I got the feeling from John that it was ultimately up to me but that he hoped I would be open to giving it another go. He was okay with only having one child before the second pregnancy, but since we took that step, he didn't want to go back. We knew being pregnant didn't sit well with me, and he was willing to pull a more significant load, just like last time. I, on the other hand, didn't know at all.

I received an email with the subject *32 weeks—your due date is approaching—what's on your mind?* I realized I had canceled all the doctor's appointments but failed to unsubscribe to all newsletters.

A few weeks later, I got an email from Amazon stating that someone had bought a gift from a baby registry that wasn't active. They sent another email the following day, admitting it was a mistake. I also received emails from other places with subject lines like *The baby is coming soon!* and *Has the baby arrived yet?* Unsubscribing from everything seemed like an impossible task. Every email served as a painful reminder.

We went to my coworker Melissa's wedding the following weekend. When the first person asked how I was doing, I answered, "Okay." I didn't think about my answer until afterward. We had a babysitter for Juni, and it was a nice change to spend time with other adults. The speeches started during dinner, and a flood of emotions hit me. Several speakers mentioned that Melissa had two brothers and was the only daughter. I couldn't hold back my tears. People might have thought the speeches moved me. It's difficult to describe how special occasions like these make me feel. I feel for the only daughter we have and the daughter we didn't have. For weddings we'll attend and weddings that will never happen.

Fredrik Backman's summer talk on Swedish radio moved me deeply. He talked about writing, about emotions, and that if you cry when you write, others will, too. I hoped it was true. Sometimes, my tears blurred the words, and I only hoped that my fingers found the correct keys. Backman also said that he writes everywhere, on his phone and on old envelopes. I wrote most of this book on my cell phone while tears streamed down my cheeks.

Keeping the abortion a secret was eating me up inside. I wanted to tell people to ease the burden in my heart. It wasn't easy that only those closest to me knew. It was difficult to pretend this year hadn't been one of the worst in my life. Dwelling on it was tough, but not dwelling was even tougher. Although uncertain about the how, when, or where, I couldn't stay silent much longer. I worried about the country we lived in. Even though abortion was legal, it wasn't accepted everywhere. I posted a comment about abortion on Twitter, and it received immediate attention from conservative trolls. I can only imagine the backlash I would have faced if I confessed to having an abortion myself. A small part of me wondered how acquaintances would react and what they would say. Then I thought, *Be careful what you wish for*. But we must be free to have a dialogue. Our voices must be heard.

One in four pregnancies in Sweden ends in abortion, while in the United States, one in four women will have had an abortion by age forty-five. These numbers mean that many women have had or will have an abortion, and I only knew a few. Many are likely afraid to confide in people. Some may judge themselves. Others may believe their loved ones would never make such a "foolish mistake." And many think that something like that would never happen to them. These harmful beliefs help explain the hatred and misconceptions. But in reality, there's a good chance that someone you know has had or is thinking about having an abortion, perhaps even yourself.

What would have been our due date was approaching, and it filled my mind with endless "what ifs" and thoughts of what could have been. Coping with everything was hard while living in the United States. I imagined it might have been easier in Sweden. While still heartbreaking, I would've preferred an experience without the stigma that haunted US politics. Abortion shouldn't be a taboo topic, and all emotions related to it should be accepted.

In the United States, abortions are frequently depicted inaccurately, falsely suggesting that women experience intense suffering and remorse. A doctor in San Diego even falsely claims to have invented a "reversal" procedure that he says can stop a medication abortion halfway through. The American College of Obstetricians and Gynecologists has denounced the "procedure." There is no need for this nonsensical behavior. Studies have shown that women don't change their minds. The very few who experience uncertainty are often misinformed and believe myths about abortion, such as the false link to breast cancer.

The grief we felt was unrelated to the abortion. Instead of regret, I felt an overwhelming sense of gratitude for being able to have an abortion. Looking back, John found it odd that he had ever hesitated. I would've preferred a clinic without bullet-proof windows and that my doctor wouldn't have had to worry about protests. I wish I had felt confident enough to discuss the pregnancy and our decision with family, friends, and coworkers without worrying about judgment. I wish there weren't news reports almost daily about Republicans' efforts to restrict abortion rights and access to birth control.

It was 2017, and I wished the future had looked brighter for my three-year-old daughter. Instead, the United States had a president who made me question why we didn't move back to Sweden for my family's sake. I realized my perception of Sweden was idealized after spending my entire adult life in the

United States. Still, Sweden has been a strong advocate for gender equality for a long time. It's consistently ranked as one of the best countries to be a woman and raise children in.

John's mom visited again, and I brought up the elephant in the room when we had a moment alone. "How do you feel about all that has happened? About . . . the abortion?" I asked. She looked me in the eye.

"I fully support you," she said. "And when I was expecting James, I did an amniocentesis too, and I don't know what we would have done if we had received a bad result," she continued.

I nodded before saying, "No, no one can know until you're in that awful situation." We were quiet until I said: "I wish you wouldn't have shared the pregnancy news, though."

Now, she nodded. "I know, and I'm so very sorry." It was a relief to discuss everything, knowing she truly meant what she said.

My in-laws had recently moved from Washington, DC, to Nashville, Tennessee, a considerably more conservative region. My father-in-law's sister already lived there, and she and her husband threw a cocktail party to welcome my in-laws. They invited a few of my father-in-law's former classmates from his law school days in Nashville. During the party, one of them boasted about their law firm's role in a lawsuit against Planned Parenthood. The party was in May, the same month I had my abortion. A year and a half later, in December 2018, I read that the last clinic offering abortions in Nashville had been forced to close. It broke my heart that progress went in the wrong direction and that the man at the cocktail party got what he wanted.

Our neighbor Jane texted me with the idea of organizing a baby shower for Nicole, our other neighbor who was pregnant. I hesitated. While I liked Nicole, Jane was very conservative—

she and her husband were Trump supporters. I talked to John, and he encouraged me to go. In the spring, Jane had questioned why she never saw me outside playing with Juni. I wanted to tell them about our abortion but felt sick thinking about it.

We never found out how that conversation would have ended. At least not this time, because the doctors had induced Nicole's labor, and their daughter was born the next day. The fetus had stopped moving, and the doctors wanted to be on the safe side. All ended well, and the family was back home.

I read in the newspapers that Princess Madeleine of Sweden and her husband Chris were expecting their third child. They were doing great. I wondered if any royals have had abortions and how they would receive a child with developmental disabilities. Can you become king with an extra chromosome? The birth of the heir was still seven months away. I wondered what would happen if something unexpected occurred—would an abortion be called a miscarriage? Or would the family welcome a royal baby with a chromosomal abnormality? The Royal Family support many charities for people with special needs. Yet, perspectives can differ when deciding what's best for your family.

Soon after, news broke that Catherine, Duchess of Cambridge, in the British royal family, was also pregnant. Some individuals in our friend group had also announced the same news recently. It seemed like everyone was getting pregnant. I wished that sorrow and pain were allowed to take the same place as joyful news. It didn't always feel that way.

In season four of the TV series *The Crown*, we saw how Queen Elizabeth II's two cousins, Nerissa and Katherine Bowes-Lyon, were admitted to an asylum in 1941. The facility was previously known as the "Asylum for Idiots" and the Royal Earlswood Institution for Mental Defectives, reflecting the shame and stigma surrounding individuals with mental illnesses and developmental disabilities during that time. The facility later changed its name to Royal Earlswood Hospital. Nerissa and Katherine were undoubtedly the Queen's cousins, but the truth about their mental health and the Royal Family's efforts to conceal them remains unknown. In 1987, when the public learned about the sisters' fate, Buckingham Palace issued a single statement: "We have no comment about it at all. It's a matter for the Bowes-Lyon family." I wondered how people would react to royals with chromosomal abnormalities in the present day.

My medical group organized a companywide event to boost employee morale every year. The executive leadership participated in skits, awarded prizes, and the company choir performed. Motivational speakers inspired the audience, followed by a documentary featuring real-life patient stories.

I usually enjoyed these events and would leave motivated and proud of my workplace. But this year, it felt different. When the choir came in and sang "What Are You Waiting For?" I couldn't hold back my tears. I usually got emotional seeing the patient stories in the documentary, a new one every year. This year, I was angry and disappointed instead. The medical group and its hospitals can perform extraordinary surgeries. But when I decided to have an abortion, they referred me to Planned Parenthood, forcing me to receive care behind bulletproof glass and with the blinds drawn. I was disappointed and ashamed that they couldn't—or wouldn't—give women the care we so desperately need without catering to the fear and bias of others by outsourcing the procedure. Among nearly twenty thousand employees, most were women, and many of them would have or consider having an abortion at some point in their lives. Studies indicated it was riskier to have a colonoscopy than an abortion, and the medical group performed those.

It was only then that I began to reflect on the fact that they had referred me to another organization. I returned home and couldn't stop thinking about how my medical group sent me to Planned Parenthood. During the night, I started drafting a letter to the senior leadership of my company in my mind.

September is usually one of the hottest months of the year in San Diego, and this year, it was also the month I would no longer give birth. I had a doctor's appointment booked with my primary care physician. The nurse checked my blood pressure and pulse before he arrived. She asked if I always had a high heart rate or if I was worried or sad about something, and my tears came instantly. We talked about how I felt, and she was kind and understanding. So was my doctor. My medical group provided me with exceptional care both before and after the abortion. It was still painful that they gave a referral for the abortion procedure. I wanted to ask someone how it works in Sweden, but I realized I didn't know anyone who had told me they had an abortion there.

After some internet searches, I found out that a doctor must perform abortions in Sweden and that they are typically performed at hospitals or women's clinics. While your regular doctor's office may not offer abortion services, they can still support you by providing information and connecting you with a local midwife clinic.

After a few days of consideration, I sent the following email to the CEO of the medical group:

Hello,

I have worked for this medical group since 2011 and I have attended the All-Staff Assembly every year it has been organized. Previous years I have always left the event feeling motivated, happy and proud to be working here, but this year was different for me.

Walking into the hall there were pictures of Susan B Anthony, Amelia Earhart, Marie Curie, Rosa Parks, and more. The documen-

tary showed the amazing surgeries we can provide, and the speakers and new advertising campaign stressed how every moment matters. All very impressive, yet earlier this year I was referred to Planned Parenthood for an abortion after it was discovered that the fetus had chromosomal abnormalities. While everyone at Planned Parenthood was wonderful, I had expected to receive care in one of our clinics instead.

I don't understand why my abortion was "outsourced" and I also don't know if that is the case for all patients or just some. But personally, I feel disappointed because our mission is to become the BEST place to work, practice medicine and receive care. I feel disappointed because I recently read a post on our intranet talking about how we are "daring to go beyond stigma and controversy." I feel disappointed because an organization that employs around 20,000 people, the majority women, sent me elsewhere for a procedure that many women will need, and that reportedly has a major complication rate that is lower than that of a colonoscopy. My PCP even stated what a simple procedure it really is.

I feel that a healthcare provider that is not religiously affiliated and that strives to become the BEST in the universe, should offer this procedure to the women it serves. The theme of this year's All-Staff Assembly was "Daring Greatly," and the speaker communicated that "fear can destroy optimism." So in the words of the choir, "what are you waiting for?"

I would love to hear your thoughts on this. Thank you for your time, Linda

I sent my email to the CEO of the medical group at 9:20 a.m. on September 6. Six days later, at 1:53 p.m., she called me. The conversation lasted around five minutes. I felt relieved when she contacted me, and despite her CEO-like response, she seemed to care. Her answers lacked persuasion, but I found out where she stood and what the head of obstetrics and gynecology thought. As an employee, I understood. But as a patient, I didn't understand.

She claimed the medical group didn't offer abortion services because of long wait times. She also said that when doctors are no longer required to perform a procedure, convincing them to do it again becomes challenging. I never found out if my medical group had a history of performing abortions or if they had always steered clear of them. I shared with her that my doctor had mentioned the medical group's fear of protests, but she insisted that wasn't the case. I pointed out that this behavior was inconsistent with our marketing message, which bothered me. I also mentioned that I didn't know they did referrals for abortions until right when I received one and was only told that the abortion needed to be done as quickly as possible once the decision had been made. They provided no other explanation. She said they would consider changing the referral process so patients could be better prepared, which would at least be a start.

My eyes welled up with tears, and I started hyperventilating. Although I struggled to recall all my thoughts and arguments, I got the most important things off my chest. While grateful for her call, I couldn't shake the feeling that she wanted to avoid leaving a record of our conversation.

I hadn't told our department yet, but I felt I had to do it soon.

John's part-time contract ended, so he applied for unemployment benefits. He was discouraged that he hadn't found a new job yet and realized he would have to expand his job search criteria. I thought about how different life would have been if we had continued the pregnancy. By now, I would have been on parental leave, and we would have been even more stressed about our finances. John would have had to prepare for life as a full-time stay-at-home dad, and I would have had to return to work earlier than I did when Juni was born.

I focused on work, my family, and the book. John struggled with unemployment and the Sisyphean labor of job search. He took on more responsibility for Juni, and I was the breadwinner.

A pregnant coworker and I went to a meeting at the office. Another coworker was already on parental leave. As we entered the room, a woman exclaimed, "Wow, it seems contagious." Then she asked me, "Why aren't you pregnant, too?" The question was harmless, but I could barely swallow, let alone answer. Eventually, I responded, "One at a time is enough." The meeting ended, and I wished I had told her the truth. It wasn't the first time the question had come up, and probably would not be the last. I hoped I would be better prepared next time.

Americans observe Labor Day on the first Monday in September. Our friends had decided to spend the long weekend with their families in a cabin by a lake in the mountains. John was still unemployed, and we had no money to spend on a vacation. Our friends wanted us to join them anyway and offered to let us sleep on a sofa bed. A woman in the group was 19 weeks into her pregnancy. I couldn't help but think about what I went through in week 19. We only stayed one night. I couldn't cope socially for more than a day and struggled to explain my feelings. But John understood and drove us home, even though Juni and our friends protested.

With less than two weeks to go until the estimated due date, I emailed our department at work, briefly explaining what I had been going through. There's never a right time to share this type of news, but I knew I needed to get it off my chest, although I didn't know how they would react. I paused and took a deep breath before I hit send. I wrote: *Most of you don't know I was pregnant earlier this year, but after bad news on the NIPT, confirmed by an amniocentesis, we sadly decided to terminate the pregnancy. I have wanted to share this with you for a while, but have not found the right time or place. Please feel free to talk to me about it, because I feel that so many women go through this, and yet it is not widely talked about.*

My colleague Michelle, who already knew about the abortion, answered immediately: *Thank you for being brave and sharing this Linda! I think you expressed it very well and really left the door open for people to talk to you! You are amazing!*

The next message said: *I am so sorry that you had to experience this Linda. You are right, many women go through this and while the circumstances may be different, the sadness and pain are the same. You have taken a step to create a platform for us women to be able to discuss this more openly. You are such a strong woman to be able to share your story with us—thank you!*

We spoke later, and it turned out that she had also had an abortion. I wasn't alone. It's a shared experience among many women, past, present, and future. She had her abortion at Planned Parenthood as well, but for her, it was because she didn't have health insurance at the time. It surprised her when I told her that our medical group had sent me there. We made plans to have lunch and continue our conversation another day.

My inbox pinged again. *Thank you for sharing this. I have had a few other friends go through the same and I cannot imagine all of the emotions. My husband and I are most likely going to start trying next year and I worry about many things. Thanks for letting me know you're here to talk about it and for being so brave.* I realized that most people knew someone who had an abortion and that often, if someone says they haven't, it may be because they haven't dared or wanted to share.

Another email came an hour later. *Thank you for sharing and I am so sorry you and John had to go through such a difficult situation . . . It's hard enough to suffer a miscarriage but to make a decision like you both had to, I could only imagine how difficult that must have been. I know you didn't have to share that with us so I really do appreciate you sharing. And I know we don't see each other since we are all at home, but sometimes when someone is off for a while and we know it's not because they went on vacay somewhere fun, I know for myself, I do wonder if that person is okay. I hope you and John are doing better and will not let this stop you guys from trying again. I will keep your family in my prayers.*

Another colleague wrote: *I'm truly sorry for your loss Linda. Sorry you had to go through this. It must have been a very hard decision. But only God knows why things happen. I'm sure he has something great planned for you. Thanks for sharing and I'm here if you need me.*

Some colleagues hadn't replied to my email by the end of the day, but I preferred their silence unless they had something nice to say.

I also emailed Dr. Patel, who worked closely with our department. We were going to a conference the following week, and I wanted him to know before we went. I sent him the same email that I had sent to our department. His response was short and to the point: *Linda, thank you for sharing.* While we held similar political beliefs, he typically avoided talking about personal matters.

A few days passed before I received more messages: *Thank you for sharing your story. You are right, so many women go through this and do not talk about it but I'm glad you said something. This just shows how close of a group we are and how lucky we are to be on this team. I can empathize with you on how hard of a decision it was to make and I am so sorry for your loss. I'm always here if you need anything!*

So sorry to hear. Looks like it's been a rough few months for lots of people. I hope you are doing well, and looking forward to seeing you tomorrow.

My department gathered for a team lunch at a restaurant close to my house the following day. Most of my coworkers were there. I felt relieved that I had told them and appreciated their responses. I suspected sharing my feelings was necessary for the emotional healing process.

After a weekend when John was out of town, I traveled to a work conference in Los Angeles. It was nice to escape the routine of everyday life. I arrived at the hotel a few hours earlier than anticipated. Instead of watching TV, reading a book, or getting some much-needed rest, I continued to work on my manuscript. The will to tell my story was stronger than ever.

In the evening, I had dinner with a couple of coworkers, and in the taxi on the way back to the hotel, I sat next to Dr. Patel. He commended my courage and suggested I engage in social activism, given my passion for the cause. I told him about my conversation with the CEO. Her response surprised him, but he was still glad she had gotten back to me. Having support and knowing someone was listening meant a lot to me. I had watched *The Wizard of Oz* with Juni the weekend before, and Dr. Patel's words made me feel like the lion. I hadn't considered myself brave, but maybe I was, after all.

The next day, I attended a seminar about the American opioid epidemic, which made me question why I hardly got any pain relief on the first day of the abortion. At the time, I didn't think much of it. But looking back, I wondered if it was another way of punishing women.

With less than a week to go until the estimated due date, my thoughts constantly went to what could have been if only the cells and chromosomes had done what we wanted them to. My emotions took control, overpowering logical thinking. I felt a mixture of sadness and relief about the abortion. Explaining it was tough and would be hard to understand for someone who hadn't been in the same situation. I felt grief about a situation which, in the eyes of some, I had chosen myself. But I hadn't done that. Not everyone understood that.

The week turned out to be much harder than I anticipated. I had already shed so many tears during the year. We could have welcomed a baby this week, but the reality was different. A birth involved immense physical pain, but I struggled with the emotional pain instead. What could have been. What we dreamed and hoped for. Instead, we found ourselves back at square one. Only this time, I was older, and our finances were worse. The joy in life was our daughter.

I emailed and texted our families: *It's okay to tell people about my pregnancy and that we ended it. It feels better to talk about it now so you can tell whoever you want. It's up to you.*

I also emailed friends in Sweden. *I know I've been bad at keeping in touch, especially this year, but I've had a lot to deal with. I was pregnant earlier this year, but prenatal testing (NIPT) showed that there was a risk of chromosomal abnormalities, which an amniocentesis confirmed. We decided to terminate the pregnancy. Around the same time, my mom underwent surgery, where they removed one kidney and the ureter when she was diagnosed with lymphoma. In addition, John lost his full-time job at the beginning of the year and, recently, his part-time job at the same company. As you can tell, we've had a tough year, and it's only now that I'm ready to talk about it. Everything is well with Juni; you probably see some photos on Instagram, right? Your children have grown so much; it's so fun to see their pictures. How are you all?*

As time passed, I told more and more people my story, and my heart got lighter each time. The daughter and sister, who only existed in our hearts, deserved better than our silence.

14

ESTIMATED DUE DATE

The day finally came. The estimated due date. A milestone. The day I had looked forward to and would later come to dread. There had been far too many days like that this year. I glanced down at my stomach, and while it wasn't as flat as it could have been, it was flatter than I had wished for it to be.

I knew I would feel pain, but I didn't expect this indescribable emptiness. My world felt devoid of color.

I took the day off from work, and several friends reached out to me. Sara came by with a card, a bottle of wine, crackers, and cheese. I was thankful that we had such good friends—a priceless gift.

The next day on Instagram, my feed was flooded with pictures supporting abortion rights in Sweden. On September 28, people worldwide unite to support the right to safe and legal abortion on International Safe Abortion Day. There were significantly more images with the Swedish hashtag #ståuppförabortsrätten than its English counterpart #internationalsafeabortionday. I might not have known it was today if I hadn't checked Swedish accounts and newspapers.

While browsing the images, I couldn't help but feel proud to be Swedish. The liberal abortion laws in Sweden provide a sense of security for those who posted these pictures, as they were unlikely to become targets of hate and violence. Sweden wasn't exempt from criticism, and it was also a relatively sensitive subject there. Still, I don't think anyone felt their life was in danger. The situation was different in the United States. The limited availability of books on this subject may be because of the potential for violence against authors, made worse by the lenient gun regulations in this country.

I wanted to teach Juni the value of peacefully standing up for one's beliefs. I hoped the saying "the pen is mightier than the sword" would hold true.

Jenny was ready to tell people about her miscarriage. I wondered if it was easier for her now because she was pregnant again. In her blog, Jenny openly discussed the challenges of parenting and bravely shared her story of miscarriage and the pain of silence. "Everything was perfect, but then it wasn't," she wrote. I could relate and being open about everything that had happened felt good. In the United States, criticism was a significant risk I had to be prepared for.

I went to the office downtown. As usual, finding parking was a challenge. Since I didn't have to be there at a specific time, I drove around the neighborhood until I found an open parking spot. Even though it was the end of September, it was warmer than most Swedish summer days.

My pregnancy was over. The pregnancy had ended several months ago, and even without having an abortion, it would have ended by now. I stood tall, took a deep breath, and walked toward the office building. The pavement was cracked and old, but it did its job. I would have to do my job, too.

The body has an incredible ability to heal, both mentally and physically, if we allow it. I decided to stop dwelling and let my heart work despite the hole it would always have. I would still allow myself to cry sometimes, but my focus would be on the future. My family would get extra hugs today.

The following day, I came down with a terrible cold. I was completely knocked out, and it took me over a week to recover.

On October 1, 2017, we woke up to the news that another mass shooting had taken place—this time in Las Vegas—and it was the deadliest in United States history to date. Swedish author and reporter Carina Bergfeldt wrote on Instagram: "It never gets easier. It can never be easier." Once again, it ignited a debate on gun legislation. As a Swede, I couldn't comprehend why stricter control hadn't been put in place yet.

Meanwhile, Puerto Rico was still struggling after the hurricane that had devastated large parts of the island. Amid all that, Republicans still focused their energy on trying to limit abortion rights. How could that be their priority? I couldn't take it anymore, but giving up on fighting for the right to safe and legal abortions wasn't an option.

15

ABORTIONS LATER IN PREGNANCY

M ost abortions aren't performed out of concern for the fetus or the woman's health. I belonged to the minority, alongside others who wanted children but had to make the difficult choice to have an abortion later in the pregnancy due to medical reasons.

Some politicians in the United States and Sweden are pushing to lower the legal limit for when abortions can be done, further straining an already challenging situation. Several American states already have laws where abortions are illegal after week 20. In Sweden, abortions are legal until week 18. After that, they're only permitted under specific circumstances. The Swedish Legal Counsel at the National Board of Health and Welfare makes the decision based, among other things, on the woman's age, mental health issues, or fetal abnormalities. The cutoff for abortion in Sweden is at 21 weeks and six days of pregnancy.

I had my abortion in week 19. If I had done it earlier, I wouldn't have known for sure if the fetus had a chromosomal abnormality or not. I could have had an abortion at week 11, but then I would have had to wonder for the rest of my life if the

NIPT result was correct, and I would have been devastated had it been false. Although it's preferable to have an earlier abortion, I didn't have that option.

We can only hope that as scientific research progresses, one will be able to receive a diagnosis earlier during pregnancy in the future. But right now, we need the option of abortions later in the pregnancy. The majority of abortions in Sweden are done early in the pregnancy. In 2016, 53 percent of all abortions were performed before week 7 and 94 percent before week 12. Most women who have an abortion later in the pregnancy want to keep the child, but for medical reasons, they make the heartbreaking decision to have an abortion for the good of the fetus and the family.

We saw what old acquaintances were up to on Facebook, even though we no longer had any contact. Kelly, one of John's old friends, was married to a Republican politician, and I had unfollowed her during his election campaign. John had seen her status updates until now. He reached his breaking point when she shared how she and her two young sons protested against abortion with signs that read *abortion kills children* and *Jesus forgives and heals*. I was at a loss for words. I wanted to write to her, but John stopped me. We knew it wouldn't be worth the backlash if I spoke up. But I hesitated because I wanted to stand up for my values and beliefs.

I realized that arguing was pointless. The disregard for rationality, logic, and scientific evidence by abortion opponents, particularly the religious right, made the situation seem hopeless. But facts are crucial, especially considering President Trump's hostility toward news channels and newspapers, dismissing anything unfavorable as "fake news."

There's a genre of viral videos showing children with different developmental disabilities in different scenarios. There are moments when they're inspiring, but at times, John and I can't help but question the intent behind those films. What is the purpose of creating this content? The suspicions are sometimes confirmed—John's friend Kelly would share such videos on social media to influence public opinion against abortion.

My trust in Sweden took a hit when I learned that some politicians were advocating for a ban, or at least restrictions, on the right to abortion. While not on par with the United States, it was still an alarming trend. Many people didn't understand why the limit couldn't be lowered. They argued that if you knew you were pregnant earlier, you could have an abortion earlier. That is true, but if you had done the NIPT and found out that there was a risk of a chromosomal abnormality, a diagnosis wouldn't have been possible at that point. Pregnant women deserve the right to know without making an abortion decision solely based on risk. There were many cases where amniocentesis later showed that it was a false positive result, and these women then continued their pregnancies. They might not have been willing to wait if they didn't have the option of a later abortion. Suppose the abortion limit was lowered; then those who aren't willing to have an abortion based solely on risk may ultimately be forced to give birth to children with severe health problems. I don't know what I would have done if the legislation had forced the issue, and I was grateful that I didn't have to face such a decision.

A man tweeted that you could easily limit the right to abortion with three weeks, since almost everyone knows that they are pregnant early on. He clearly didn't understand the difference between an abortion early and later in the pregnancy. The ignorance behind such claims is astounding.

Fetal anomalies and chromosomal abnormalities can rarely be confirmed until later in the pregnancy. If the test results had been different, some of us who have abortions might have chosen to keep the fetus. Would the abortion opponents rather have an abortion at week 10, when there is still a chance that the fetus is healthy? The answer is evident: they don't want us to have abortions at all.

Planned Parenthood organized a conference called the *Goodbye Stigma Summit* in San Diego, and I decided to go. The day before the conference, I received an email from the organization warning that protesters would most likely be there, and they asked all conference attendees to ignore them. The notice said the protesters love to argue and asked all attendees to walk by quietly and calmly regardless of what they may be shouting. The email also mentioned that there would be bag checks for everyone entering as an extra security measure. I had to admit I was nervous. There were no protesters outside the abortion clinic when I was there, but that was more the exception than the rule. I also thought about how often shootings occur in this country.

I parked in the parking garage next to the hotel overlooking the harbor. When I walked into the lobby, I didn't see anyone wearing the iconic pink "I Stand With Planned Parenthood" shirt. Planned Parenthood wasn't listed on the hotel's notice board with all the conferences. It was already 1:00 p.m.; check-in had started fifteen minutes ago, and the event was beginning in half an hour. I took the escalator to the floor with all the conference rooms but couldn't find the right place.

Was it the wrong date? I double-checked my ticket, and it confirmed that it was the right day. Despite wandering around, I still couldn't locate the conference. I returned to the lobby and walked up to the information desk. After I asked where the Planned Parenthood conference was held, the man behind the counter took out a calendar. He didn't find anything, so I asked for the *Goodbye Stigma Summit* instead. He had to ask his manager, who then directed me to the part of the hotel I should go to. They didn't want to advertise Planned Parenthood's presence—another security measure.

I took the escalators back up to a secluded part of the hotel, where I finally glimpsed some people in pink shirts. There were no signs, no information to show the way. I approached the check-in desk and saw armed security guards stationed on both sides. They asked for my ID and gave me a purple wristband that I had to wear for the entire conference. They searched my purse, and I went through a metal detector to get to the conference rooms. A leaflet was distributed to all participants, urging us to inform the security guards if we noticed anything suspicious, saw participants without wristbands, or felt threatened or unsafe. I had butterflies in my stomach, and they weren't the good kind.

The goal of the conference was to give the participants the knowledge to help reduce the stigma that surrounds abortion in our society. The event had plenty of inspiring speakers who shared my perspective on abortion, which I found incredibly meaningful.

Although many participants had undergone abortions, none of them mentioned having done it for medical reasons. I wish I could have had the chance to talk to someone who could relate to my situation.

16

PREGNANT?

I was overjoyed when my parents finally came to visit from Sweden. Given my mom's surgery earlier in the year, I was especially thrilled this time. It was a relief that she was healthy enough to travel. Juni hadn't seen them in over a year, so I wasn't sure how she would react, but as soon as they arrived, she examined them with her doctor's toys—she approved.

It dawned on me a few days later that my period was overdue. I checked the period tracker app on my phone and confirmed that my period was late. After the abortion, my body hadn't been itself, and my cycle hadn't been as reliable as before when I usually knew exactly what day it would come. It had never taken this long before. We had used protection, so pregnancy was unlikely, but nothing was certain.

We all went to a fantastic seafood restaurant overlooking the harbor and downtown for lunch. Still, I could barely eat anything. Before we went, I had told John about my period being late. We didn't know what to do—should we take a pregnancy test or let the uncertainty eat at us for a while longer? I wasn't ready to be pregnant again.

We returned home, and I couldn't stop thinking about it. Was I pregnant? It should have been impossible, but my period still hadn't come. I would probably have to take that pregnancy test. I wanted it to be negative, but I didn't know if I would be disappointed if it was. If the test was positive, I would worry. Worry about how I would feel, how everything would go considering the previous pregnancy, and our finances. John had recently had a promising interview, but a week later, he still hadn't heard back.

John had planned to pick up Sara and her family at the airport late in the evening, and I asked him to buy a pregnancy test. I didn't sleep well and lay there thinking about the possibilities. One second, I was sure I was pregnant—everything I had read suggested that. The next second, I wasn't so sure. Was I feeling anxiety or nauseous? Shortly after 5:00 a.m., I needed to go to the bathroom. John had put the pregnancy test and a yellow plastic cup on the counter. He woke up and asked if I was ready. I nodded and fumbled away the plastic around the package. After 20 seconds of performing the test, I put the top back on the pregnancy test stick and waited. I had specifically asked for a test where the answer was in writing rather than lines or a plus sign.

When the answer finally came, I felt a mix of worry and relief.

The test spelled out: *Not pregnant.*

I exhaled. We hadn't planned to try, and we had used protection. But I worried. It was 35 days since my last period, and after the abortion, it had come every 24 days. Previously, my period always arrived on time every 28 days. I wondered what was happening with my body. I thought about contacting my doctor but decided I would wait another week.

My period finally came, two weeks late, along with severe cramps. I took painkillers and made the most of the last days of my parents' visit. In two days, they were set to fly back to Sweden.

The day of their departure came, and I wished they didn't have to leave. Saying goodbye was difficult. After we dropped them off at the airport, the lump in my throat grew to the point where I couldn't stop my tears. On the way home, Juni asked if I missed my mom and dad, and I replied I did, but since we lived in different parts of the world, we had to go through this.

After numerous internet searches, I found the book *Our Heartbreaking Choices*, edited by Christie Brooks. My tears came as soon as I read the dedication on the first page: "This book is dedicated to all of the women and men who have had to make the heartbreaking choice to end a much-wanted pregnancy due to a fetal anomaly or a complication with the mother's health" and "to our sweet angels."

In the book, forty-six women shared their stories of having abortions for medical reasons. The book resonated with me and sparked a deep sense of recognition. I could have written so many descriptions of events and feelings myself. I realized I wasn't alone but that so many of us who have gone through the same or similar things felt alone. Some women couldn't bring their partners into the examination room at all, some had to drive hundreds of miles for the abortion, and some had to deliver the dead fetuses. I wouldn't have been able to do that. I know we can handle things we never thought were possible, but I wouldn't have wanted to. My surgical abortion was painful enough.

I received an email from an organization for chromosomal abnormalities seeking volunteers for their research studies. The list of different research studies was long—all the complications that could happen seemed endless. It certainly wasn't something I would have wished for our child.

17

A NEW CHAPTER

F all passed, and John and I were frustrated that he no longer had a job. We sometimes discussed another attempt to expand the family, and John said he wanted to but preferred to have a job first. I wasn't sure that my body could adapt to that timeline. After my parents' visit, I knew I wanted to wait until after Thanksgiving in late November when John's family would come to visit. But if we were to try, it had to be shortly afterward. I didn't want to give birth after I turned forty, so we only had a window of a few months.

I turned to the internet to find out the risk of a chromosomal abnormality in a new pregnancy. It depended on the type of abnormality. The risk was low if unrelated to any hereditary problem, which was the case for us. My age posed a bigger problem.

Was I ready to be pregnant again? Absolutely not. Was I scared and worried about what would happen if I got pregnant again? Absolutely.

John's family came to visit, and like most American families, we enjoyed a traditional Thanksgiving meal with turkey, potatoes, green beans, cranberry sauce, and my favorite, stuffing.

We celebrated at our house because John's family had thought we would have a newborn baby, and it would have been easier for us not to travel. Although we didn't have a baby, the plans remained, and everyone gathered here for the long weekend. Juni appreciated the company and the attention. I struggled with emotions I hadn't expected would emerge around the holidays—still, the thoughts of what could have been. The only person who mentioned it to me was Megan, my sister-in-law. I was grateful she didn't ignore what happened and understood I wanted to discuss it.

A month passed, and as Christmas approached, I painfully realized how different my family and life were from what I had imagined. John had a seasonal job over the holidays, often leaving me alone, and I spent much of that time crying. I didn't want to spoil the Christmas joy for my family and friends, so I suffered alone. The year had been horrible beyond comprehension, an ordeal I wouldn't wish on anyone. The things that brought brightness to my life were my daughter, husband, dog, parents, and closest friends. I don't know what I would have done without them. I counted the days until this nightmare year, our annus horribilis, would end.

As the year was coming to an end, we decided not to use birth control anymore. It was with mixed feelings, and I hoped it wasn't a decision we would regret. We had to see if my body would cooperate or not. There were no guarantees; we knew that all too well.

This year was cursed. We knew that reality wasn't a fairy tale and that most people didn't live happily ever after, but I sincerely hoped that the upcoming year would be better for our family.

I still felt sad thinking about how different our family could have been by now. When I looked at the ultrasound pictures from the second pregnancy, my grief overwhelmed me.

However, I could also find happiness in spending time with our family—I could smile, play with Juni, and enjoy the present. I hadn't made it to acceptance, but I now thought there was a possibility that one day I would.

The bells rang in the new year, and we left 2017 behind. With a kiss to my husband and a hug to our sleeping daughter, we closed that chapter. A new chapter was on the horizon, and with it, the potential for something good, something better. My wish this time was for a book with a happy ending.

The new year started with John accepting a job offer he had received. His first day as a project manager for a defense contractor was in February. By then, I realized my period was late once again. It had been unpredictable after the abortion, so maybe it didn't mean anything. The pregnancy test I had ordered the day before was waiting in the bathroom. I waited for John to come home from work to take it. I should have been preparing dinner, but I couldn't focus. Some of Juni's preschool friends had become big sisters and brothers, so she asked if I had a baby in my belly and said she wanted a little sister. I answered truthfully that I didn't know and that there was no way to decide if it would be a sister or a brother.

Somehow, I managed to make dinner, and it was ready when John came home. We ate, and I drank glass after glass of water. When dinner was over, I walked upstairs to our bathroom and peed in the plastic cup I had set out earlier.

A few minutes later, the test showed the result.

I was pregnant.

I had suspected it, since I was so tired, and a touch of nausea had crept up on me during the day. My feelings were mixed. This time, I wasn't nearly as sure that we would have a baby in the end.

After a few days, the shock subsided, and a more intense realization and fear set in. Tears, which hadn't been as frequent lately, returned in a flood. We were filled with both happiness and fear, worried that the nightmare from the year before would be repeated. But all I could do was make my doctor appointments and hope for a better year. From the bottom of my heart, I wished the chromosomes wouldn't play tricks on us. I hoped we would never, ever have to stand on the other side of the bulletproof glass again.

18

OUR RAINBOW CHILD

I read Hillary Rodham Clinton's book *What Happened*, where she expressed a frustration I could relate to. She wrote that she had lost count of the times she had been sitting at her kitchen table working on her book when a breaking news alert interrupted her. She had hung her head, sighed, and then had to take out the red pen and start revising. Abortion rights were a constant topic in the United States, so I repeatedly experienced that same feeling.

President Trump's nomination of Judge Brett Kavanaugh to the Supreme Court raised concerns about the future of abortion rights. Kavanaugh's well-documented opposition to abortion sparked worries that he would favor overturning *Roe v. Wade*. Given his views on women, it also wasn't surprising that he faced sexual abuse accusations.

In the end, it didn't matter. Christine Blasey Ford's courageous testimony failed to persuade the Supreme Court, and they swore in Brett Kavanaugh as a Supreme Court justice. My heart stung. The idea of my daughter having to live in a country without abortion rights was beyond imagination. This looming reality and many decisions made by Trump and the Republicans made the future look darker than it had in a long time. Most parents had lived with the hope and faith that their children would be better off than themselves. Unfortunately, at least in the United States, that trend seemed to have reversed.

The abortion issue was also a topic in the Swedish election debate. We must never take the right to legal and safe abortion for granted, and we must continue to talk about abortion and normalize it as a fundamental part of women's healthcare.

The debate will no doubt continue worldwide after I complete this book. However, I'll continue to share my experiences and fight for my children to grow up in a world where no one questions the right to abortion.

I was understandably nervous when I sat in the lab to do the NIPT test again. The nurse about to take the blood sample asked, "What do you want it to be?"

I looked at her and answered, "Healthy." She continued to pressure me about what sex I wanted the fetus to be until I burst into tears, and other staff entered the room wondering what was going on. I told them I had done the same test the year before and received devastating news and that I had had an abortion after an amniocentesis confirmed the result. Hopefully, the nurse will treat other patients with more empathy in the future and not assume the woman is there to find out the sex of the fetus. You can do the test for more than one reason.

When I left, she said, "I'll pray for you."

We didn't have to return to Planned Parenthood.

Ludvig, our healthy baby boy, was born in late 2018. Tears flowed down my cheeks as I held him tightly in my arms. The journey leading to this moment had been an emotional roller coaster. A piece of my heart would always be reserved for my unborn daughter, but the rest belonged to my family. My family was complete now. Welcome, our rainbow child.

EPILOGUE

Midsummer is my favorite Swedish holiday; it's such a happy time. Nothing compares to those nights when the sun barely sets. My social media feed usually fills with idyllic pictures, which makes me sad when I'm not in Sweden celebrating with family and friends.

On Midsummer's Eve in 2022, I was scrolling through pictures on Instagram as the news hit—the Supreme Court had overturned *Roe v. Wade*. There had been rumors that this would happen after the Supreme Court draft opinion leaked in May 2022, but I didn't want to believe it could happen. But it did. All the fears I had voiced in this book had become reality. My social media feed became an absurd mix of happy Midsummer celebration pictures mixed with the gut-wrenching news that the Supreme Court's ruling had struck down the constitutional right to abortion in the United States.

Three days later, the Swedish edition of this book was scheduled to be published. The timing was eerie, and I posted a picture of myself on Instagram wearing a T-shirt with the text *Bans off our bodies*. I captioned it: "I'm mad and sad, and let my shirt speak for me. On Monday you can buy my book where I share what it was like to have an abortion in the United States." It was a marketing opportunity I wished I hadn't had.

At the end of 2022, twelve states were enforcing a near-total ban on abortion with few exceptions. I can only hope that I'll write another epilogue for a future edition of this book where I can share how abortion is safe, legal, and accessible in all states in the United States and around the world. Until then, we need to talk about abortion and stand up for abortion rights everywhere.

SOURCES

Books

Bengtsdotter, A. (2017). *100 om dagen: berättelser om abort*. Leopard förlag.

Bergfeldt, C. (2019). *Tre dagar med Ku Klux Klan*. Tiden.

Brooks, C. (2008). *Our Heartbreaking Choices: Forty-Six Women Share Their Stories of Interrupting a Much-Wanted Pregnancy*. iUniverse, Inc.

Clinton, H.R. (2017). *What Happened*. Simon & Schuster UK.

Delaney, J.P. (2017). *The Girl Before*. Ballantine Books.

Grimes, D.A. & Brandon, L.G. (2014). *Every Third Woman in America: How Legal Abortion Transformed Our Nation*. Daymark Publishing.

Hjort, P. (2013). *Missfall: med rätt att sörja*. Vulkan.

Junger, S. (2016). *Tribe: On Homecoming and Belonging*. Hachette Book Group.

Kondo, M. (2017). *Konsten att städa: förenkla ditt liv med ett organiserat hem*. Pagina Förlags AB.

Ohlsson, K. (2019). *The Flood*. Simon & Schuster UK.

Sandell, Å. (2016). *Den tuffaste ronden: en personlig historia om abort, missfall, IVF och äggdonation*. Kalla kulor förlag.

Tännsjö, T. (1991). *Välja barn: om fosterdiagnostik och selektiv abort*. Bokförlaget Thales.

Articles

1177 Vårdguiden. (2015). *Vad är fosterdiagnostik?* Retrieved September, 26, 2017, from https://www.1177.se/barn--gravid/graviditet/undersokningar-under-graviditeten/fosterdiagnostik/

1117 Vårdguiden. (2015). *Fostervattensprov*. Retrieved November 12, 2017, from https://www.1177.se/barn--gravid/graviditet/undersokningar-under-graviditeten/fostervattenprov/

Ansari, A. & Croffie, K. (2017, January 9). *Kentucky abortion bills signed, effective immediately*. CNN. Retrieved October 28, 2017, from http://www.cnn.com/2017/01/08/us/kentucky-abortion-bills-pass/index.html

ANSIRH. (2017, 29 mars). *TV greatly exaggerates the medical and psychological risks associated with abortion*. Retrieved November 12, 2017, from https://www.ansirh.org/research/research/tv-greatly-exaggerates-medical-and-psychological-risks-associated-abortion

Australian Breastfeeding Association. (2015). *Rapid weaning (Lactation suppression)*. Retrieved October 30, 2017, from https://www.breastfeeding.asn.au/bfinfo/lactation-suppression

Babycenter. (2008-2017) *Termination for Medical Reasons: Public Group*. Retrieved October 30, 2017, from https://community.babycenter.com/groups/a6325/termination_for_medical_reasons

Bowman, E. (2017, March 18). *Wisconsin Upsets NCAA Defending Champions Villanova*. NPR. Retrieved October 29, 2017, from http://www.npr.org/sections/thetwo-way/2017/03/18/520675445/wisconsin-upsets-ncaa-defending-champions-villanova

Brownwyn, I. (2017, May 11). *The Power Of The Word "Abortion"*. Bustle. Retrieved December 8, 2017, from https://www.bustle.com/p/the-power-of-the-word-abortion-55737

Callstam Jörnmark, D. (2017, April 7). *Stockholmare svarar på attacken med kärlek och pizza*. Aftonbladet. Retrieved December 8, 2017, from https://www.aftonbladet.se/nyheter/godanyheter/a/G70A4/stockholmare-svarar-pa-attacken-med-karlek-och-pizza

Campoamor, D. (2018, March 26). *Abortion AMA: Can My OB/GYN Provide An Abortion?* Bustle. Retrieved February 9, 2019, from https://www.bustle.com/p/abortion-ama-can-my-ob-gyn-provide-abortion-8538823

Campoamor, D. (2018, November 9). *GOP opposition to birth control is politics, period*. CNN. Retrieved January 12, 2020, from https://www.cnn.com/2018/11/

09/opinions/contraceptive-mandate-alabama-west-virginia-abortion-campoamor/index.html

Caplan-Bricker, N. (2015, November 30). *Attacks on Abortion Clinics Should Be Prosecuted as Terrorism.* SLATE. Retrieved January 26, 2018, from http://www.slate.com/articles/double_x/doublex/2015/11/attacks_on_abortion_clinics_should_be_prosecuted_as_terrorism.html

Cha, A.E. (2018, March 5). *Babies with Down syndrome are put on center stage in the U.S. abortion fight.* The Washington Post. Retrieved January 9, 2019, from https://www.washingtonpost.com/news/to-your-health/wp/2018/03/05/down-syndrome-babies-are-taking-center-stage-in-the-u-s-abortion-fight/?noredirect=on&utm_term=.24cc471ca504

Chappel, B. (2017, October 25). *'Jane Doe' Immigrant Has Abortion In Texas, After Battle With Trump Administration.* NPR. Retrieved October 30, 2017, from http://www.npr.org/sections/thetwo-way/2017/10/25/560013894/jane-doe-has-abortion-in-texas-after-battle-with-trump-administration

Chuck, E. (2018, June 5). *What is Roe v. Wade? Everything you need to know.* NBC News. Retrieved February 15, 2019, from https://www.nbcnews.com/storyline/smart-facts/what-roe-v-wade-everything-you-need-know-n856891

Cohen D.S. (2017, April 19). *Bill O'Reilly's Dangerous War Against Dr. Tiller.* Rolling Stone. Retrieved January 26, 2018, from https://www.rollingstone.com/politics/features/bill-oreillys-dangerous-war-against-dr-tiller-w477824

Crockett, E. (2017, January 12). *The GOP's crusade to defund Planned Parenthood nationwide, explained.* Vox. Retrieved October 30, 2017, from https://www.vox.com/identities/2017/1/12/14189500/defund-planned-parenthood-congress-paul-ryan-republicans

Dayton, T. (2017, March 31). *Why We Grieve: The Importance of Mourning Loss.* Huffington Post. Retrieved January 12, 2018, from https://www.huffingtonpost.com/entry/why-we-grieve-the-importance-of-mourning-loss_us_58de79c6e4b0d804fbbb7226

Dube, R. (2017, May 10). *A message for mothers with an aching heart, on Mother's Day.* TODAY. Retrieved October 28, 2017, from https://www.today.com/parents/message-mothers-aching-heart-mother-s-day-t111228

Eaton, B. (2017, October 3). *33, Married, & Ready For A Baby: I Am The Face Of*

Late-Term Abortion. Refinery29. Retrieved January, 27, 2018, from http://www. refinery29.com/2017/07/162888/second-trimester-abortion-personal-experi ence?utm_source=email&utm_medium=email_share

Flury, A. (2017, October 30). *US abortion doctor says 'I'm not going to live in fear'*. BBC. Retrieved January 26, 2018, from http://www.bbc.com/news/world-us-canada-41525400

Foley, E. & Reilly, R. (2017, October 25). *'Jane Doe' Got Her Abortion. Trump Policy Will Still Block Them For Other Immigrant Teens*. Huffington Post. Retrieved February 9, 2019, from https://www.huffingtonpost.com/entry/undocu mented-teen-abortion_us_59ef98a9e4b0bf1f883676c2

Franchell, E. (2017, October 17). *Ebba Busch Thor smyger om aborterna*. Afton-bladet. Retrieved October 30, 2017, from https://www.aftonbladet.se/ledare/ a/pJWK1/ebba-busch-thor-smyger-om-aborterna

Glenngård, A. (2020, June 5). *International Health Care System Profiles: Sweden*. The Commonwealth Fund. Retrieved November 3, 2023, from https://www. commonwealthfund.org/international-health-policy-center/countries/ sweden

Glenza, J. (2019, July 25). *Doctor claiming to 'reverse' abortion was told to stop using medical school's name*. The Guardian. Retrieved November 3, 2023 from https://www.theguardian.com/world/2019/jul/25/revealed-doctor-reverse-abortion-trump-administration

Graham, R. (2017, July 18). *A New Front in the War Over Reproductive Rights: 'Abor-tion-Pill Reversal'*. The New York Times Magazine. Retrieved January 21, 2018, from https://www.nytimes.com/2017/07/18/magazine/a-new-front-in-the-war-over-reproductive-rights-abortion-pill-reversal.html

Grönlund, E. (2018, February 7). *Experten: "Målet med fosterdiagnostik är inte att Downs syndrom ska minska"*. SVT. Retrieved February 16, 2018, from https:// www.svt.se/nyheter/vetenskap/experten-malet-med-fosterdiagnostik-kan-inte-vara-att-down-syndrome-ska-minska

Gunter, J. (2017, December 10). *Abortion: Separating fact from harmful fiction*. Marin Independent Journal. Retrieved January 27, 2018, from http://www. marinij.com/health/20171210/abortion-separating-fact-from-harmful-fiction

Hansson, F. (2017, March 20). *Rocka sockorna! Därför bär vi omaka strumpor*.

Expressen. Retrieved September 29, 2017, from http://www.expressen.se/ halsoliv/manskligt/rocka-sockorna-darfor-bar-vi-omaka-strumpor/

Hay, L. & Kessler, D. (2015, February 6). *The 3 Most Devastating Kinds Of Loss (And How To Recover)*. Huffington Post. Retrieved December 8, 2017, from https:// www.huffingtonpost.com/2015/02/06/recover-from-devastating-loss_n_6608514.html?ncid=engmodushpmg00000006

Haynes, D. (2014, December 9). *Abortion complication rates are 'very low,' study says*. UPI. Retrieved December 8, 2017, from https://www.upi.com/ Health_News/2014/12/09/Abortion-complication-rates-are-very-low-study-says/3591418165114/

Johnson, T.M. (2016, May 17). *Coping with Grief and Depression After an Abortion*. PsychCentral. Retrieved December 8, 2017, from https://psychcentral.com/ lib/understanding-abortion-grief-and-the-recovery-process/?all=1

Kaposy, C. (2018, April 16). *The Ethical Case for Having a Baby With Down Syndrome*. The New York Times. Retrieved January 9, 2019, from https:// www.nytimes.com/2018/04/16/opinion/down-syndrome-abortion.html

Krajewski, C. (2017, July 10). *I used to be quiet about the fact that I perform abortions. Now I'm upfront*. The Washington Post. Retrieved January 26, 2018, from https://www.washingtonpost.com/news/soloish/wp/2017/07/10/i-perform-abortions-the-men-i-date-often-see-me-as-a-political-symbol/?utm_cam paign=healthfb&utm_content=content2-october17&utm_medium=post& utm_source=facebook&utm_term=.28c8obd13101

Lussenhop, J. (2015, September 25). *What is Planned Parenthood*. BBC. Retrieved February 16, 2019, from https://www.bbc.com/news/world-us-canada-34363358

Magnegård Bjers, C. (2005, May 16). *Var fjärde graviditet slutar i abort*. Aftonbladet. Retrieved January 21, 2018, from https://www.aftonbladet.se/ wendela/article10596832.ab

March of Dimes. (2016). *Genetic Counseling*. Retrieved October 5, 2018, from https://www.marchofdimes.org/pregnancy/genetic-counseling.aspx

Menza, K. (2017, May 24). *Dirty Dancing Is, Was, and Will Forever Be a Movie about Abortion*. Harper's BAZAAR. Retrieved January 6, 2018, from http://www. harpersbazaar.com/culture/film-tv/a9924985/dirty-dancing-remake-abortion/

National Society of Genetic Counselors. (2018). *Find a Genetic Counselor.* Retrieved October 5, 2018, from https://www.nsgc.org/page/whoaregcs

Olsson, A. (2017, April 12). *Barnmorskan som vägrar abort förlorade i Arbetsdomstolen.* Vårdfokus. Retrieved September 29, 2017, from https://www.vard fokus.se/webbnyheter/2017/april/barnmorskan-som-vagrar-abort-forlorade-i-arbetsdomstolen/

Pearson, C. (2017, April 6). *The Most Outrageous Abortion Legislation Of The Last Month.* Huffington Post. Retrieved October 9, 2018, from https://www.huffing tonpost.com/entry/the-most-outrageous-abortion-legislation-of-the-last-month_us_58e3e9f2e4b0f4a923b2bd22

Pehrson, L. (2012, January 27). *Nya lagar inskränker rätten till abort i USA.* Sydsvenskan. Retrieved October 30, 2017, from https://www.sydsvenskan.se/2012-01-27/nya-lagar-inskranker-ratten-till-abort-i-usa

Petterson, L. (2018, February 7). *Färre barn föds med Downs syndrom i Sverige – fler aborteras.* SVT. Retrieved December 12, 2018, from https://www.svt.se/nyheter/vetenskap/farre-barn-fods-med-downs-syndrom-i-sverige-fler-aborteras

Planned Parenthood. (2017). *In-Clinic Abortion.* Retrieved October 28, 2017, from https://www.plannedparenthood.org/learn/abortion/in-clinic-abortion-procedures

Planned Parenthood. (2019). *This is Who We Are.* Retrieved February 16, 2019, from https://www.plannedparenthood.org/uploads/filer_public/a0/96/a09686b9-1fb2-4b37-96c7-4a874a44d22b/190117-whoweare-factsheet-v01.pdf

Planned Parenthood. (2017). *What happens during an in-clinic abortion?* Retrieved November 12, 2017, from https://www.plannedparenthood.org/learn/abortion/in-clinic-abortion-procedures/what-happens-during-an-in-clinic-abortion

Planned Parenthood. (2017). *Who We Are.* Retrieved October 30, 2017, from https://www.plannedparenthood.org/about-us/who-we-are

Pålsson, C. (2019, June 29). *Abortdebatt pressar KD i opinionen: "Begränsat till det".* Di. Retrieved January 31, 2020, from https://www.di.se/nyheter/abortdebatt-pressar-kd-i-opinionen-begransat-till-det

Quinones, J. & Lajka, A. (2017, August 15). *"What kind of society do you want to live in?": Inside the country where Down syndrome is disappearing.* CBS News. Retrieved January 21, 2018, from https://www.cbsnews.com/amp/news/down-syndrome-iceland/

Rankin, L. (2017, August 16). *Abortion on TV and in Movies Is Way Too Dramatic — Here's Why. Allure.* Retrieved January 12, 2018, from https://www.allure.com/story/abortion-on-tv-and-movies-is-too-dramatic/amp

Ravitz, J. (2016, June 27). *The surprising history of abortion in the United States.* CNN. Retrieved March 10, 2019, from https://www.cnn.com/2016/06/23/health/abortion-history-in-united-states/index.html

Region Stockholm. (2020). *Abort.* Retrieved February 8, 2020, from https://www.barnmorskemottagningar.se/graviditet/oonskad-graviditet/

RFSU. (2017, September 27). *Imorgon tar världen ställning för aborträtten.* Retrieved January 12, 2018, from https://globalportalen.org/artiklar/imorgon-tar-varlden-stallning-for-abortratten

Richards, C. (2014, October 16). *Ending the Silence That Fuels Abortion Stigma.* ELLE. Retrieved October 28, 2017, from http://www.elle.com/culture/career-politics/a15060/cecile-richards-abortion-stigma/

Roberts, M. (2017, October 4). *Yes, Rep. Tim Murphy is a hypocrite on abortion. That's not the worst part.* The Washington Post. Retrieved October 9, 2018, from https://www.washingtonpost.com/blogs/post-partisan/wp/2017/10/04/the-gop-rep-who-asked-his-mistress-to-get-an-abortion-might-still-think-hes-pro-life/?noredirect=on&utm_term=.e1fef5b449fb

Rochman, B. (2017, August 19). *The disturbing, eugenics-like reality unfolding in Iceland.* QUARTZ. Retrieved January 21, 2018, from https://qz.com/1056810/the-disturbing-eugenics-like-reality-unfolding-in-iceland/

Russonello, G. (2017, May 2). *Jimmy Kimmel's Emotional Monologue: His New Son's Heart Condition.* The New York Times. Retrieved September 29, 2017, from https://www.nytimes.com/2017/05/02/arts/television/jimmy-kimmel-baby-son-wife.html

Rydhagen, M. (2017, October 23). *"Bebisluckorna är ett otroligt korkat förslag".* Expressen. Retrieved October 30, 2017, from https://www.expressen.se/kvallsposten/bebisluckorna-ar-ett-otroligt-korkat-forslag/

Sacchetti, M. & Marimow, A.E. (2017, October 20). *Appeals court delays abortion for undocumented teen; gives government time to find her a sponsor.* The Washington Post. Retrieved October 30, 2017, from https://www.washingtonpost.com/local/immigration/appeals-court-weighs-whether-immigrant-teen-can-be-denied-abortion-while-in-us-custody/2017/10/20/ab414d2a-b50c-11e7-9e58-e6288544af98_story.html?utm_term=.7809c43f07e4

Siddiqui, S. (2018, January 18). *How has Donald Trump's first year affected women?* The Guardian. Retrieved February 9, 2019, from https://www.theguardian.com/us-news/2018/jan/18/how-has-donald-trumps-first-year-affected-women

Sifferlin, A. (2017, October 3). *This Is How Far American Women Have to Travel to Get an Abortion.* TIME. Retrieved January 12, 2018, from http://time.com/4967735/how-far-american-women-travel-for-abortion/

Socialstyrelsen. (2016, November 14). *Kromosomavvikelser, en översikt.* Retrieved January 11, 2019, from https://www.socialstyrelsen.se/kunskapsstod-och-regler/omraden/sallsynta-halsotillstand/kromosomavvikelser-en-oversikt/

Socialstyrelsen. (2017, July 12). *Spinal muskelatrofi.* Retrieved January 11, 2019, from https://www.socialstyrelsen.se/kunskapsstod-och-regler/omraden/sallsynta-halsotillstand/spinal-muskelatrofi/

Spychalsky, A. (2017, September 14). *7 Low-Key Horrifying Things Women Have Been Subjected To In 2017.* Bustle. Retrieved February 9, 2019, from https://www.bustle.com/p/these-2017-attacks-on-womens-rights-are-difficult-to-relive-2351028

Stone, M. (2017, July 27). *What It Was Like to Be an Abortion Provider in the U.S. Before Roe v. Wade.* TIME. Retrieved January 26, 2018, from https://time.com/4873317/abortion-provider-interview/

Svensk Förening för Medicinsk Genetik och Genomik. (2018). *Genetiska vägledare.* Retrieved October 5, 2018, from https://sfmg.se/sfmg/om-klinisk-genetik/genetiska-vagledare/

SVT. (2017). *Fakta: Det här gäller för abort i Sverige.* Retrieved January 27, 2018, from https://www.svt.se/nyheter/inrikes/fakta-det-har-galler-for-abort-i-sverige

Uffalussy, J.G. (2017, June 7). *Here's the Cost of an Abortion: Different Types, Insur-*

ance Plans, and More. Glamour. Retrieved October 5, 2018, from https://www.glamour.com/story/how-much-does-an-abortion-cost

Vincenty, S. (2021, November 23). *All About Nerissa and Katherine Bowes-Lyon, the Queen's Hidden Cousins.* Oprah Daily. Retrieved April 1, 2021, from https://www.oprahdaily.com/entertainment/tv-movies/a34576867/queen-elizabeth-hidden-cousins-nerissa-katherine-bowes-lyon/

Wadhwani, A. (2018, December 10). *Planned Parenthood, the only abortion provider left in Nashville, suspends abortion services.* Nashville Tennessean. Retrieved February 8, 2019, from https://www.tennessean.com/story/news/2018/12/10/planned-parenthood-nashville-abortion-clinic/2266196002/

Winkley, L, Kucher, K. & Figueroa, T. (2017, May 1). *Poolside party becomes 'war zone' as gunman shoots seven, is killed by cops.* The San Diego Union-Tribune. Retrieved October 30, 2017, from http://www.sandiegouniontribune.com/news/public-safety/sd-me-shooting-universitycity-20170430-story.html

Wright, J. (2017, June 19). *Why A Pro-Life World Has A Lot of Dead Women In It.* Harper's Bazaar. Retrieved January 26, 2018, from http://www.harpersbazaar.com/culture/features/a10033320/pro-life-abortion/

Zachariasson, H. (2017, March 24). *Trump drar tillbaka sin sjukvårdsreform.* SVT Nyheter. Retrieved October 28, 2017, from https://www.svt.se/nyheter/utrikes/trumps-sjukvardslag-har-inte-tillrackligt-med-roster

Radio

Backman, F. (2017, July 30). *Sommar & Vinter i P1.* Retrieved October 28, 2017, from http://sverigesradio.se/sida/avsnitt/921590?programid=2071

Film/TV

(2017) *Korrespondenterna* [TV program]. SVT. https://www.svtplay.se/korrespondenterna

Ardolino, E. (Director). (1987). *Dirty Dancing* [Film]. Great American Films Limited Partnership, Vestron Pictures.

Bicks, J. (Writer), Frankel, D. (Director). (2001, August 5). *Sex and the City: Coulda, Woulda, Shoulda* [TV program]. Darren Star Productions.

Chupack, C. (Writer), Engler, M. (Director). (2004, January 18). *Sex and the City: Catch-38* [TV program]. Darren Star Productions.

Crane, D. (Writer), Kauffman, M. (Writer), Bilsing, S. (Writer), Kreamer, E. (Writer), & Halvorson, G. (Director). (2004, February 19). *Friends: The One Where Joey Speaks French* [TV program]. Bright/Kauffman/Crane Productions/Warner Bros. Television.

Fleming, V. (Director). (1939). The Wizard of Oz [Film]. Metro-Goldwyn-Meyer (MGM).

Handler, C. (2017, June 1). *Chelsea: Changing the Climate* [TV program]. Netflix.

Meyers, N. (Director, Writer). (2006). *The Holiday* [Film]. Columbia Pictures/Universal Pictures/Relativity Media/Waverly Films.

Shane, M. (Director, Writer), Wilson, L. (Director, Writer), O'Toole, G. (Writer). (2013, January 18). *After Tiller* [Film]. Code Red Pictures/Artemis Media Ventures/Belle Max Productions/Chicken And Egg Pictures.

Songs

"Better Place (Tille's Song)", Camilla Gervide, 2006

"Some Die Young", Laleh, 2012

Other References

Gervide, C. (2017, March 22). *Rocka sockorna eller?* Retrieved October 30, 2017, from https://nyheter24.se/bloggbevakning/2017/03/22/rocka-sockorna-eller/

Nash, E., Gold, R.B., Mohammed, L., Ansari-Thomas, Z. & Cappello, O. (2018, January 2). *Policy Trends in the States, 2017.* Guttmacher Institute. Retrieved January 28, 2018, from https://www.guttmacher.org/article/2018/01/policy-trends-states-2017

Nash, E. & Guarnieri, I. (2023, January 10). *Six Months Post-Roe, 24 US States Have Banned Abortion or Are Likely to Do So: A Roundup.* Guttmacher Institute. Retrieved April 30, 2023, from https://www.guttmacher.org/2023/01/six-months-post-roe-24-us-states-have-banned-abortion-or-are-likely-do-so-roundup

Persson, K. (2017, October 18). *Begränsa aborträtten med tre veckor....är det något att bråka om..man vet väl mkt tidigare att man är gravid......* [Twitter post]. Retrieved January 12, 2018, from https://twitter.com/ganterud/status/920562220794368000

Slack2thefuture. (2017, January 27). *Remember sitting in history, thinking "If I was alive then, I would've..." You're alive now. Whatever you're doing is what you would've done.* [Twitter post]. Retrieved January 12, 2018, from https://twitter.com/slack2thefuture/status/825198136071032832

ACKNOWLEDGMENTS

Thank you to my daughter. You're the sunshine in my life. You're my everything. I love you.

Thank you to my son. You made our family complete. You're our rainbow child. I love you.

Thank you to my husband. No one should have to experience what we went through, but if you must, I wish everyone a husband like you. You were there to hold my hand when the tears wouldn't stop, through all the grief and pain, and when I wanted to tell the world. Thank you for always listening, for your support, and for loving me. I love you.

Thank you to my parents for always loving me, no matter what. I love you.

Thank you to my beloved dog, Leia. You gave me more than eleven years of unconditional love. You were always faithfully there, putting your head in my lap and licking my tears. I miss you more than any words can describe. I love you.

Thank you to my best friends for always being there and listening to me. I appreciate your friendship more than you will ever know. You know who you are. I love you.

Thank you to everyone who keeps fighting for the right to abortion to remain (or become) a reality. We need you.

Thank you to all the doctors, nurses, and staff who are working in abortion clinics. I hope it will become easier for you as you work in the United States and other countries where opposition and hate are a part of your reality every day.

Thank you to the doctors and nurses who took care of me.

Thank you, Planned Parenthood. I will be forever grateful for the care you gave me when my medical group didn't provide me with the basic healthcare that all women should have access to.

Thank you to all women who have had a similar experience. You're stronger than you think you are, and you're not alone.

Thank you to everyone who has helped me in this book's journey to publication and the marketing following it. Thanks to you, this book can reach people and help others in the same situation feel less alone.

Thank you for reading this book.

ABOUT THE AUTHOR

Linda Rönn, originally from Sweden, traded cold winters for the sunny shores of Southern California, where she now lives with her family. A voracious reader and introvert, she finds solace and inspiration in quiet moments. Her debut book, *Behind Bulletproof Glass*, offers a unique perspective on abortion rights in the United States.

facebook.com/lindaronn.author

x.com/lindaronn

instagram.com/_lindaronn

goodreads.com/lindaronn